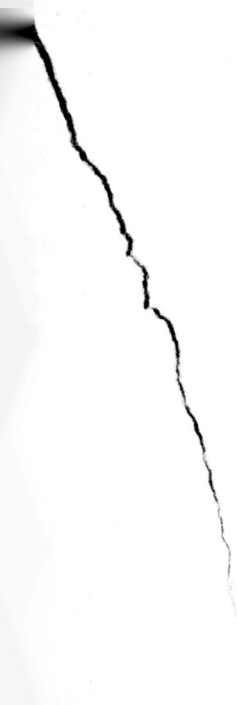

Type 3 Diabetes: The Hidden Link Between Blood Sugar, Brain Health, and Healing Naturally

Dr. Constance Santego

Maximillian Enterprises
Kelowna, BC

Type 3 Diabetes

Copyright © 2025 by Dr. Constance Santego.

Copy Editor & Interior Design: Constance Santego
Book Layout: ©2017 BookDesignTemplates.com

Ordering Information:
Quantity sales. Special discounts are available on quantity purchases by corporations, associations, and others. For details, contact the "Special Sales Department" at the address above.

Trade Paperback ISBN: 978-1-990062-81-0
Ebook ISBN 978-1-990062-82-7
Created and published In Canada. Printed and bound in the United States of America

First Edition
Published by Maximillian Enterprises
Kelowna, BC
Canada
www.constancesantego.ca

Dedication

To every soul who has ever felt the confusion of cravings, the fog of fatigue, the fear of memory slipping away, or the loneliness of waking in the night unsure of what your body is trying to tell you — this book is for you.

I dedicate these words to the countless people living with diabetes, known or hidden, and to those who love them. May you find hope, clarity, and healing here.

To my husband, who has witnessed my struggles with patience and love, and to my family who has supported me on this journey.

And to all who are seeking the true *sweetness of life* — may you discover that it is not found in sugar, but in balance, joy, connection, and peace.

"Find sweetness in your life, not just on your tongue." — *Louise Hay*

ALSO BY DR. CONSTANCE SANTEGO

NOVELS

Illegitimate Grace
Ashcroft Hollow

Okanagan Trilogy:
Beneath the Vineyards
Under the Okanagan Sun
Guardian of the Lake

The Nine Spiritual Gifts Series:
Journey of a Soul – (Vol 1 Michael)
Language of a Soul – (Vol 2 Gabriel)
Prophecy of a Soul – (Vol 3 Bath Kol)
Healing of a Soul – (Vol 4 Raphael)
Miracles of a Soul – (Vol 5 Hamied)
Knowledge of a Soul – (Vol 6 Raziel)
Wisdom of a Soul – (Vol 7 Uriel)
Faith of a Soul – (Vol 8 Pistis Sophia)

NONFICTION
The Intuitive Life, The Gift Of Prophecy, Third Edition
Fairy Tales, Dreams And Reality... Where Are You On Your Path?
Second Edition
Your Persona... The Mask You Wear
Archangel Michael's Soul Retrieval Guide
Tesla And The Future Of Energy Medicine
Beyond Tesla: Advancing The Science Of Energy Healing
Tesla's Code: Mastering Energy, Frequency, And Creative Power
Beyond The Mind: Harnessing The Power Of Astral Projection For
Creative Awakening
Bend, Don't Break: Finding Your Way Back To Abundance
Ring Therapy: A Guide To Healing And Balance
Ring Therapy Pocket Guide
Floraopathy™: The Art And Science Of Vibrational Healing With
Essential Oils
Dear Older Me: A Memoir... Of Sorts
It's Just Like Poker: A Spiritual Guide To Playing The
Cards Life Deals You
Signs And Meanings: What The Feet Reveal About Health, Stress,
And The Body's Story
Auricions: Unlocking Subconscious Healing Through Quantum
Medicine
Quick Fix Acupressure Method

REIKI WISDOM, SERIES:
Angelic Lifestyle, a Vibrant Lifestyle
Angelic Lifestyle 42-Day Energy Cleanse
Reiki and the Power of The Joint Points: Unlocking Energy Pathways
for Healing (Vol I)
Reiki and Karmic Healing: Releasing Patterns From Past Lives (Vol II)
Reiki and the Five Elements (Vol III)
Secrets of a Healer, Magic Of Reiki
The Reiki Master's Manual

SECRETS OF A HEALER, SERIES:
Magic Of Aromatherapy (Vol I)
Magic Of Reflexology (Vol II)
Magic Of The Gifts (Vol III)
Magic Of Muscle Testing (Vol IV)
Magic Of Iridology (Vol V)
Magic Of Massage (Vol VI)
Magic Of Hypnotherapy (Vol VII)
Magic Of Reiki (Vol VIII)
Magic Of Advanced Aromatherapy (Vol IX)
Magic Of Esthetics (Vol X)
The Reiki Master's Manual (Vol XI)

ADULT COLORING JOURNALS
SERIES-ZEN COLORING:
Quantum Energy and Mindful Living Journal (Vol 1)
Reiki Energy Journal (Vol 2)
Nine Spiritual Gifts Journal (Vol 3)
I Forgive Journal (Vol 4)

FOR CHILDREN
I am Big Tonight. I Don't Need the Light

COOKBOOK
My Favorite Recipes, with a Hint of Giggle

BUISNESS
How To Use Chatgpt For Authors: From Idea To Published Book
Scaling Beyond 6 Figures: Strategies For Health & Wellness
Professionals
The Academypreneur's Playbook: Turn Knowledge Into A
Revenue-Generating School

Contents

Preface

This book was born from both science and lived experience. For years, I knew something in my body was out of balance, even when the doctors' numbers said otherwise. The vivid dreams, the nighttime "episodes," the shakiness, the foggy days when words slipped away — these were the body's whispers, long before a blood test confirmed diabetes.

When I finally learned that high and unstable blood sugar doesn't just affect the body — it affects the brain — everything clicked. Suddenly, the strange link between my dreams, my moods, my memory, and my sugar levels made sense. And I realized I wasn't alone. Millions of people are living with the same condition, often undiagnosed or misunderstood.

Scientists are now calling this connection **Type 3 Diabetes** — the brain's version of diabetes, linked to memory loss, Alzheimer's, dementia, and cognitive decline. The name may be new, but the symptoms are not: brain fog, cravings, mood swings, restless nights, and early memory lapses. These are the red flags that tell us the brain is starving for balanced fuel.

This book is not about fear — it is about empowerment. You will find here both my story and the science explained simply. You'll discover foods, herbs, rituals, and practices that stabilize blood sugar, protect the brain, and restore energy. You'll learn how stress, sleep, and emotions influence sugar as much as food. And you'll see how modern medicine, ancient traditions, and lifestyle choices together create hope for healing.

My wish for you is simple: may these pages help you listen more closely to your own body's signals, nourish both your pancreas and your mind, and rediscover the true sweetness of life — the kind that comes not from sugar, but from clarity, balance, and joy.

With love and healing,
Dr. Constance Santego

Note to Reader

This book is written to educate, inspire, and empower — but it is not meant to replace medical advice. Everyone's body is unique, and diabetes shows up differently in each person. Please use these pages as a guide alongside, not instead of, the care you receive from your healthcare providers.

If you are currently taking medication for diabetes or any other condition, do not stop or adjust it without professional guidance. Some of the foods, herbs, or lifestyle practices in this book can interact with medications. When in doubt, bring this book with you to your next appointment and discuss what resonates with your doctor, naturopath, or healthcare team.

More importantly, remember this: **you are not your diagnosis.** Blood sugar imbalances and memory lapses do not define you — they are signals, not sentences. Your body and brain are asking for balance, and you have the ability to answer that call in small, powerful ways each day.

Take what serves you, experiment gently, and be patient with yourself. Some changes will feel natural; others may take practice. Healing is not a straight line. It is a rhythm — a dance between science, spirit, and self-awareness.

My hope is that these pages give you both practical tools and emotional comfort. May you walk away with not only knowledge, but also renewed faith in your body's capacity to heal and in your spirit's right to experience joy, clarity, and the true sweetness of life. Shift happens…Create magic!

How to Use This Book

This book is more than information — it is an invitation to explore, reflect, and take action. Blood sugar balance, especially when connected to brain health, can feel overwhelming. My goal is to make it simple, practical, and empowering for you.

Here's how you can get the most from these pages:

1. READ IN ORDER — OR CHOOSE WHAT SPEAKS TO YOU

The chapters build on each other, moving from my story, to science explained simply, to practical lifestyle strategies. But you don't have to read straight through. If you're drawn to food, start with Part III. If sleep and dreams are your struggle, skip ahead to those chapters. Let curiosity guide you.

2. PAUSE & REFLECT

You'll find **reflection prompts, journaling questions, and meditations** woven throughout the book. Don't rush past them. These moments are where knowledge becomes wisdom. Take a pen, jot down your thoughts, or simply close your eyes and breathe with the guidance on the page.

3. TRY, TEST, AND TRACK

Every body is unique. What balances one person may not work the same way for another. Use the food strategies, herbal suggestions, and lifestyle tools as experiments. Pay attention to how your body responds. A simple journal — even a few notes each day — will help you see patterns and progress.

4. BRING IT INTO YOUR REAL LIFE

Healing is not about perfection — it's about practice. Try one new breakfast idea. Take a short walk after dinner. Swap a sugary drink for cinnamon tea. Every small choice is a step toward balance. Don't wait for "the perfect time" — begin where you are, with what you have.

5. PARTNER WITH YOUR CARE TEAM

This book does not replace your doctor. Bring what you learn here into your conversations with your healthcare providers. Share your questions. Ask for the lab tests listed. Think of this book as a companion guide that helps you become an active, informed partner in your care.

Remember: Healing Type 3 Diabetes is not only about controlling blood sugar — it's about reclaiming the sweetness of life, protecting your brain, and rediscovering joy. Read with an open heart, and let these pages become both a map and a mirror for your own healing journey.

Type 3 Diabetes: The Hidden Link Between Blood Sugar, Brain Health, and Healing Naturally

Dr. Constance Santego

WHY DIABETES DOESN'T DEFINE YOU

Diabetes is something you live with — it is not who you are.

You are not your lab numbers, your medications, or your diagnosis. You are the person who still laughs at a joke, hugs a loved one, dreams about the future, and finds joy in the small moments. Diabetes is a condition of the body, but it does not touch the core of your spirit.

Yes, it requires awareness and care. But it also calls forth your strength, resilience, and wisdom. Every balanced meal, every mindful breath, every choice to move your body is proof that you are not powerless. You are responding. You are healing.

Your worth is not measured in A1c levels or blood sugar readings. It is measured in the love you give, the light you share, and the way you keep showing up for yourself — even on the hard days.

Diabetes may be part of your story, but it will never be your whole story.

Part I – My Story, Wake-Up Call

The Night My Body Told the Truth

It started in the dark hours of the night, when most people expect only the comfort of dreams. For me, the dreams came— but they carried something else with them. Something that jolted me awake, left me breathless, and filled my body with a kind of electric panic I didn't yet have a name for.

At first, I thought they might be panic attacks. I would wake suddenly, heart racing, lungs gasping for air as though I had just been pulled from underwater. My husband would tell me afterward that I made strange sounds, almost like a gasp mixed with a cry, sometimes so intense he said it sounded like an orgasm. The episodes lasted only seconds—ten, maybe thirty at the most—but they drained me completely. By the time the shaking and breathlessness passed, I felt as though I had run a marathon in my sleep.

The dreams themselves were vivid, almost too vivid— fragments of memory, strange flashes of thought, even moments from my childhood that hadn't surfaced in decades. They came like messengers, but what they were telling me was unclear. All I knew was that each episode left me more unsettled than the last.

During the day, I wasn't spared either. The attacks began creeping into my waking hours. My chest would tighten, my breathing would hitch, and my whole body would feel the ripple—down to my toes. At times, I wondered, *Am I dying? Is this my heart?*

Finally, fear overcame stubbornness. I went to the emergency room. That's when the truth surfaced.

After hours of tests and monitoring, a nurse came back with the numbers that changed everything: my blood sugar was 31. I was in a dangerous state, teetering on the edge where confusion, seizures, even coma were possible. Over the next seven hours, I was given multiple injections—insulin, one shot after another, in my hip. Slowly, carefully, they pulled me back from the brink.

That night was my body's wake-up call. It was as if my system had been shouting for years in whispers—through the shaky hands at eighteen, through the pre-surgery nurse's raised eyebrow at forty-five, through the cravings, the fatigue, the fuzzy vision. But I hadn't listened. Or perhaps, I hadn't understood what it was saying. Now, my body had spoken in a way I couldn't ignore.

The truth was undeniable: I had diabetes.

And yet, in many ways, this was only the beginning of my story.

REFLECTION PROMPTS

- What signals has your body given you that you may have overlooked?
- If you trace your health story back, what early clues might you now recognize?

What Most People Don't Know—Type 3 Diabetes

When I walked out of the hospital that morning, exhausted but alive, I thought the hardest part was behind me. My doctor prescribed medication, explained how to monitor my blood sugar, and assured me that with a few changes, I could get things under control.

But what no one told me—and what very few people seem to know—is that diabetes is not just about blood sugar. It's not just about the pancreas, or insulin, or numbers on a glucose monitor. It is also about the brain.

That's where the phrase **"Type 3 Diabetes"** comes in.

Most people have heard of **Type 1** diabetes, where the body doesn't produce insulin at all. They know about **Type 2**, where the body makes insulin but resists its effects, leading to chronically high blood sugar. But few people have heard of **Type 3 Diabetes**—a term that scientists and doctors increasingly use to describe the link between diabetes and Alzheimer's disease, dementia, and cognitive decline.

THE SUGAR–BRAIN CONNECTION

Here's the simple truth: your brain is fueled almost entirely by glucose. It's your most energy-hungry organ. But when blood sugar is unstable—too high, too low, or wildly fluctuating— your brain feels it first.

- That "foggy" feeling after a sugar crash? That's your brain starved of fuel.
- That sudden irritability or panic? That's glucose swinging out of range.

- Those vivid dreams and strange nighttime episodes I experienced? My brain was sounding the alarm.

When blood sugar stays high for too long, insulin resistance develops—not just in muscles and fat cells, but in the brain itself. Over time, the brain struggles to absorb and use glucose. Neurons weaken. Memory falters—mood shifts. Connections break down. This is why some researchers now call Alzheimer's **"Type 3 Diabetes."**

MY PERSONAL CLUES

Looking back, I can see the hints were there all along. The shakiness at eighteen wasn't just "nerves." The strange taste that creeps into my mouth when my blood sugar is high isn't random—it's my brain registering overload. Those vivid dream episodes weren't just panic attacks—they were signals that my brain was under stress.

The tragedy is how often these early warnings are ignored, brushed aside, or misdiagnosed. And the cost is enormous. Millions of people live with diabetes or prediabetes and never realize that their mental clarity, their memory, even their personality may be at risk.

WHY SO MANY ARE UNDIAGNOSED OR MISDIAGNOSED

One of the most dangerous truths about diabetes is how silent it can be. Millions of people live with prediabetes or undiagnosed diabetes, never realizing that their headaches, anxiety, or brain fog are part of a bigger picture.

Often, these symptoms get mislabeled:

- Anxiety or panic disorder.
- Depression.
- Stress or "burnout."
- Even just "getting older."

Meanwhile, blood sugar imbalance quietly damages the brain, the heart, the eyes, and the nerves. By the time someone is officially diagnosed, years—or decades—of damage may already be in place.

WHY THIS MATTERS TO YOU

You may be reading this because you already know you have diabetes. Maybe you take medication. Maybe you've felt the side effects I did—digestive issues from metformin, hair loss from newer drugs, or simply the exhaustion of trying to balance numbers that never seem to cooperate.

Or maybe you're here because you've started noticing things:

- Crashing in the afternoon.
- Sudden brain fog.
- Trouble remembering words.
- Strange dreams or restless nights.
- A creeping sense that something isn't right.

This book is for you.

Because once you understand that blood sugar is not just about avoiding complications "someday," but about protecting your brain, your energy, and your very sense of self—**everything changes.**

THE ROAD AHEAD

In the next chapters, I'll show you what I wish someone had told me earlier:

- The symptoms you can spot before it's too late.
- The natural ways to stabilize blood sugar and protect your brain.
- How medication and lifestyle can work together.
- And most importantly, how to take your power back—so you never feel trapped in fear the way I did that night in the hospital.

This is not just a story about diabetes. It's a story about remembering who you are, protecting your future, and giving your body and brain the balance they deserve.

Part II – Understanding Blood Sugar & the Brain

The Sugar–Brain Connection

The first thing I learned after my diagnosis was that blood sugar is about much more than numbers on a chart. It's about the way every cell in your body receives and uses energy—especially the cells in your brain.

Your brain runs almost entirely on glucose. Even though it makes up only about 2% of your body weight, it uses about 20% of your daily energy. Every thought you think, every memory you recall, every word you speak is powered by sugar molecules being burned for fuel.

So what happens when that sugar isn't handled properly?

WHEN SUGAR SPIKES – THE PREDIABETES CLUES

When you eat something sweet—or a meal full of refined carbs like white bread, pasta, or sugary drinks—your blood sugar rises quickly. Your pancreas responds by releasing insulin, the hormone that helps shuttle sugar into your cells to be used for energy.

But if your body is becoming resistant to insulin (as happens in prediabetes and Type 2 diabetes), the sugar doesn't move into the cells efficiently. Instead, it lingers in your bloodstream. You may not see the damage right away, but your brain and body *feel* it in real time.

Here's what it can look like:

- Blurred vision
- Headaches
- Brain fog or confusion
- Irritability or mood swings

And here's what it *felt like for me* before anyone ever told me the word "diabetes":

- At **nineteen**, when I was finally old enough to drink, I was what people called a "cheap drunk." One rye and ginger ale, and I'd be tipsy, far more than anyone else at the table. If I used Coke instead of ginger ale, the next morning was brutal—headache, nausea, and that sick, heavy feeling (a hangover) after only *one drink.* The only cure I ever found? A McDonald's Egg McMuffin and hashbrown to soak it up. Looking back, my body wasn't just reacting to alcohol—it was reacting to the sugar spike.
- In my **forties**, I remember a student of mine looking at me after lunch one day and asking, "What did you eat for lunch? You seem drunk?" I was stunned. The only thing I had eaten was spaghetti. What she was seeing was me riding the blood sugar high and crash.
- Another time, out at a pub with my husband and a friend, the friend asked me, "How much have you had to drink already?" I hadn't had any alcohol at all—I was drinking iced tea. What he noticed was how sugar made me act: lightheaded, almost giddy, like I was tipsy without touching a drop.

At the time, I laughed it off. But these were not random quirks. They were signs that my blood sugar was out of balance—that my brain was being flooded and then starved of energy over and over again.

Over time, consistently high blood sugar is like flooding your brain's delicate wiring system. The connections short-circuit, the lights flicker, and your clarity fades. What I thought was "just how my body reacted" was really my brain trying to cope with years of hidden prediabetes.

WHEN SUGAR CRASHES – THE HIDDEN LOWS

On the other hand, if your blood sugar drops too low—because you skipped a meal, exercised hard, or took too much medication—your brain is suddenly starved of fuel. And when the brain doesn't have enough fuel, it panics. Symptoms come fast and hard:

- Shakiness
- Sweating
- Panic or anxiety
- Sudden, urgent hunger
- Trouble thinking clearly

For years, I lived with these symptoms without knowing what they really meant.

I was always a **nine o'clock bedtime girl**. Even as a teenager, while my friends stayed up late, I'd be exhausted by nine. I remember one night when my cousin and his friends came over, and we were playing *Dungeons & Dragons*. Right at nine, I told them I had to go to bed. They probably thought I was being boring, but the truth was I could barely focus—I was drained, my concentration blurred, and my eyesight seemed to fade. I thought it was because of my vision (I lost sight in my left eye as a baby and always blamed everything on "bad eyesight"). In reality, my brain was running out of fuel.

Even into adulthood, this pattern followed me. My husband still jokes that I can fall asleep in seconds. He'll say, "I was just talking to you when you lay down," but I'd already be out cold before he finished the sentence. That instant exhaustion wasn't just a personality quirk—it was my body shutting down when my blood sugar crashed.

But the biggest red flag came in the form of **shakiness and sudden, urgent hunger.** My hands would tremble, my heart would pound, and panic would set in. My husband called it being "hangry" (hungry + angry). But to me, it felt like survival—like I *HAD* to eat something right then, or I would unravel. And the truth is, I wasn't just being dramatic. My body was sounding an emergency alarm: feed me, fuel me, or I can't function.

Looking back now, I can see that my so-called quirks—going to bed early, falling asleep instantly, getting irrationally hangry—were really blood sugar crashes. They weren't just inconveniences. They were warnings. My brain was crying out for balance, long before I ever knew the word *diabetes.*

INSULIN RESISTANCE IN THE BRAIN

Here's the part few people realize: insulin doesn't just work in your muscles and fat tissue. It works in your brain, too. Neurons (your brain cells) need insulin to pull glucose inside and use it for fuel.

When the brain becomes resistant to insulin, it's like locking the door and leaving the lights off. The fuel is right there in the blood, but the cells can't access it. Over time, this starves your neurons, damages connections, and makes memory, focus, and learning harder.

This is why researchers call Alzheimer's disease "Type 3 Diabetes." It's not just about age or genetics—it's about years of blood sugar imbalance wearing down the brain's ability to function.

THE EVERYDAY CLUES

You don't need a lab coat to notice when your brain is being affected by sugar swings. The clues are often hiding in plain sight:

- Mid-afternoon brain fog that clears up after a snack.
- Trouble remembering names or simple words.
- Cravings that feel almost irresistible.
- Sudden irritability or feeling "hangry."
- Strange dreams or restless nights.

These aren't just quirks of aging or personality. They are signs that your brain is riding the blood sugar rollercoaster.

BRAIN FOG – WHEN BLOOD SUGAR CLOUDS THE MIND

One of the most frustrating—and sometimes frightening— symptoms of blood sugar imbalance is **brain fog.** It's not a medical term, but it perfectly describes the feeling: as if your mind is wrapped in cotton, your thoughts are slow, and your memory is slippery.

I've lived this more times than I can count.

- **Mixing words or letters:** Even when I was younger, I noticed moments where I'd mix the first letters of words when speaking. It wasn't constant, but when it happened, it left me feeling embarrassed and confused. Now I understand it wasn't clumsiness—it was my brain struggling with unstable fuel.
- **Forgetting why I walked into a room:** After I had children, I began to notice a new pattern. I would walk

into a room and completely forget why I was there. I'd have to retrace my steps, go back to where I started, and try to jog my memory. At the time, I brushed it off as "mom brain," but now I know better.

- **Losing my train of thought mid-sentence:** More recently, I've noticed that if I get interrupted while speaking, I sometimes completely lose track of what I was going to say. The thought is just gone. This isn't only about distraction—it's about blood sugar swings interfering with the brain's ability to hold and retrieve information.

WHY BRAIN FOG HAPPENS

Your brain is a glucose hog. It uses more sugar than any other organ. When blood sugar spikes and then crashes, your neurons lose their steady fuel supply; it's like flickering electricity: one minute the lights are bright, the next they dim or go out.

- **High blood sugar** overwhelms neurons, making signals sluggish.
- **Low blood sugar** starves them, making memory and focus unreliable.
- **Insulin resistance in the brain** means even when sugar is available, cells can't use it well.

The result: word mix-ups, memory lapses, mental fatigue, and that frustrating "Why did I come in here?" moment.

THE EMOTIONAL TOLL

Brain fog doesn't just affect thinking—it affects confidence. I used to wonder if I was scatterbrained, careless, or even showing early dementia. But once I realized these were blood sugar signals, not character flaws, it gave me both relief and motivation.

The same way blood sugar swings create brain fog, stabilizing your meals, sleep, and stress can clear it. Balanced meals keep glucose steady, hydration helps neurons fire properly, and daily movement increases blood flow to the brain.

When you protect your blood sugar, you don't just protect your body—you keep your mind sharp, your words clear, and your memory intact.

THE TASTE–MEMORY LINK

One of the strangest but most consistent clues I've had is a **taste in my mouth that comes with a memory or daydream.** It's hard to describe—almost metallic, almost sweet—but it's unmistakable.

What I've since learned is that blood sugar affects neurotransmitters—the chemical messengers in the brain that shape mood, memory, and focus. When glucose is high or low, it can change the way these neurotransmitters fire. That's why a memory might be triggered at the same moment you sense a taste, or why a daydream can carry a physical flavor.

It's not just "in your head." It's the chemistry of your brain reacting to changes in blood sugar.

THE BIG PICTURE

Too high, and your brain is flooded. Too low, and it's starved. And when insulin resistance develops in the brain, neurons slowly wither from lack of fuel.

That's the sugar–brain connection in its simplest form. And it's why blood sugar balance is not just about avoiding diabetes complications. It's about protecting your most precious organ— your brain.

THE HOPEFUL NEWS

Here's the part that gives me hope—and should give you hope too: just as quickly as blood sugar can go out of balance, it can begin to stabilize when you make changes. Every balanced meal, every walk after dinner, every night of good sleep helps your brain regain some of its resilience.

Blood sugar balance is brain balance. Protect your blood sugar, and you protect your memory, your clarity, and your future self.

REFLECTION PROMPTS

- When was the last time you felt brain fog or a memory slip? What was happening with food, stress, or sleep around that time?
- Do you notice a taste, dream, or body sensation that warns you your sugar is high or low?

The Nerve Sheath & Brain Health

(Why Blood Sugar Affects Memory, Mood, and Cognition)

1. WHAT IS THE NERVE SHEATH (MYELIN)?

- Each nerve in your brain and body is like an electrical wire.
- To work properly, that wire needs insulation — this insulation is called the **myelin sheath.**
- Myelin is made of fat and protein, wrapping around nerves to make signals fast and clear.
- Healthy myelin = sharp thinking, stable mood, quick reflexes.
- Damaged or thinned myelin = brain fog, memory lapses, slower thinking, mood swings, and even nerve pain.

2. THE BLOOD SUGAR LINK

- Chronically high blood sugar causes **inflammation and oxidative stress** that damage myelin.
- Excess sugar also attaches to proteins and fats in the brain (glycation), making the myelin stiff and dysfunctional.
- Insulin resistance (Type 2 & Type 3 diabetes) reduces the brain's ability to use glucose efficiently, essentially "starving" neurons despite sugar flooding the blood.
- Over time, this contributes to:
  - **Alzheimer's disease** (often called "Type 3 Diabetes").
  - **Dementia** and memory decline.
  - **Cognitive impairment,** such as brain fog, word mix-ups, and poor focus.

3. MYELIN & TEENAGERS (WHY GRADE 9 FEELS LIKE A TURNING POINT)

- During childhood, the brain is actively building myelin — the "insulation" that helps nerve signals travel quickly and smoothly.
- Around ages **12–16**, especially during the middle-to-high school transition, the brain enters a phase of **pruning and remodeling.** Instead of shedding myelin, the brain is:
    o Strengthening the connections that are used most often.
    o Letting go of unused connections.
    o Re-myelinating key pathways for efficiency.
- During this remodeling, communication between brain regions can feel slower or less consistent, which may show up as:
    o Mood swings, irritability, or impulsiveness.
    o Forgetfulness or trouble focusing.
- Combined with powerful hormonal changes, this brain remodeling explains much of the emotional turbulence in adolescence.
- By the late teens and early twenties, the prefrontal cortex (the "logic and decision-making" center) becomes more fully myelinated, supporting **clearer thinking, better focus, and steadier emotional regulation.**

4. THE DIABETES–DEMENTIA–MYELIN TRIANGLE

- **Unstable blood sugar** in youth may disrupt myelin development, making mood swings worse.
- **Chronic high blood sugar** in adulthood accelerates myelin damage, brain aging, and memory loss.
- **Balanced blood sugar** across life: protects myelin, sharpens memory, stabilizes mood.

5. SUPPORTING MYELIN HEALTH

- **Balanced blood sugar:** stable glucose prevents glycation and oxidative damage.
- **Healthy fats:** omega-3s (salmon, walnuts, flax, chia), olive oil, coconut oil = building blocks of myelin.
- **B vitamins:** especially B12 and folate, crucial for myelin repair.
- **Movement:** exercise increases blood flow to the brain, nourishing myelin.
- **Sleep:** myelin repair happens most during deep sleep.
- **Gut health:** a healthy microbiome reduces inflammation that otherwise strips myelin.

Key Takeaway:
The **myelin sheath is the insulation for your brain's wiring.** Blood sugar swings damage it, while stable glucose protects it. That's why diabetes, Alzheimer's, and dementia are linked — they all involve **myelin breakdown.** And just like teenagers experience mood swings during myelin remodeling, adults with unstable blood sugar experience brain fog, memory slips, and emotional volatility.

Signs & Symptoms You Should Never Ignore

For years, I brushed off the signs my body was giving me. I thought I was just tired, stressed, or maybe "wired differently." In truth, my body had been waving red flags all along. The problem was, I didn't know what those flags meant.

Blood sugar imbalances don't always show up as obvious "diabetes symptoms." They sneak in through everyday moments—moments you may have already experienced yourself.

THE SUBTLE BUT SERIOUS CLUES

Here are some of the most common ways blood sugar instability shows itself:

- **Shakiness**: trembling hands, weak knees, or feeling jittery for no clear reason.
- **Cravings**: especially for sugar or carbs, soon after eating.
- **Sudden hunger**: that desperate "I need food right now or I'll fall apart" feeling.
- **Vision changes**: blurriness that comes and goes with blood sugar shifts.
- **Panic or anxiety**: feelings that come out of nowhere, sometimes mistaken for a mental health condition.
- **"Dream episodes"**: vivid dreams or night terrors, waking up gasping, trembling, or drenched in sweat.
- **Strange tastes or sensations**: metallic, sweet, or bitter tastes that show up during memories, daydreams, or moments of brain fog.
- **Exhaustion**: needing to sleep early, crashing after meals, or falling asleep the instant your head hits the pillow.

- **Brain fog**: difficulty concentrating, forgetting words, or feeling like your thoughts are moving through molasses.
- **Mood swings**: irritability, feeling "hangry," or emotional swings that don't match the situation.

YOUR SELF-AWARENESS CHECKLIST

Take a moment to reflect. How many of these sound familiar to you?

- Do you get shaky, sweaty, or lightheaded if you miss a meal?
- Do you crave sweets or carbs even after you've just eaten?
- Do you ever feel drunk or giddy without drinking alcohol?
- Do you experience panic or a racing heart at night?
- Do you feel tired all the time, no matter how much sleep you get?
- Have people ever asked if you're "on something" when you've just eaten sugar or carbs?
- Do you notice blurred vision that comes and goes?
- Do you fall asleep almost immediately when you lie down?
- Have you ever had vivid dreams or night episodes with gasping, trembling, or strange sounds?
- Do you experience brain fog, trouble focusing, or memory lapses?

If you checked several of these boxes, it may be more than just stress or "getting older." These can be early warning signs of blood sugar imbalance—and sometimes, undiagnosed diabetes.

WHEN TO SEEK MEDICAL HELP IMMEDIATELY

While many blood sugar swings can be managed with lifestyle changes, there are times when you should not wait:

- If your blood sugar (with a home monitor) is consistently above 200 mg/dL (11 mmol/L) or below 70 mg/dL (3.9 mmol/L).
- If you faint, have seizures, or experience severe confusion.
- If you have chest pain, shortness of breath, or dizziness with high/low blood sugar episodes.
- If you wake repeatedly at night with panic, trembling, or gasping.
- If you notice sudden changes in vision, especially blurriness or dark spots.

These symptoms can indicate dangerously high or low blood sugar and require immediate medical care.

THE KEY TAKEAWAY

The earlier you catch these signs, the easier it is to restore balance. Don't wait until your body is screaming at you the way mine did. Pay attention to the whispers—the cravings, the exhaustion, the hangry moments—because those whispers are the beginning of your body's story.

Your Pancreas, Your Powerhouse

Most of us go through life without giving our pancreas a second thought. It's a small organ, about six inches long, tucked behind your stomach. But this quiet little organ is one of the hardest-working heroes in your body—and when it struggles, everything else does too.

WHAT THE PANCREAS ACTUALLY DOES

Think of your pancreas as both a chef and a traffic controller:

1. **As a chef** – it releases digestive enzymes into your intestines to help you break down fats, proteins, and carbs. Without it, your body couldn't fully digest food.
2. **As a traffic controller** – it monitors the amount of sugar (glucose) in your blood. When glucose rises after a meal, your pancreas sends out **insulin** to help shuttle that sugar into your cells for energy. When glucose dips, it releases **glucagon**, which tells your liver to release stored sugar and keep your energy steady.

This constant balancing act keeps you alive, fueled, and thinking clearly.

WHEN THE SYSTEM BREAKS DOWN

There are different ways the pancreas and insulin system can falter:

- **Type 1 Diabetes** – the pancreas stops making insulin altogether because the immune system attacks the insulin-producing cells. Without insulin, glucose can't get into cells at all.
- **Type 2 Diabetes** – the pancreas is still making insulin, sometimes even *too much*, but your cells have become

resistant to it. The pancreas gets overworked trying to
keep up, and eventually, it may tire out.

- **Prediabetes** – somewhere in between. The pancreas is
producing insulin, but not enough to keep up with the
resistance in the cells. Blood sugar climbs silently, often
for years, before symptoms are obvious.
- **Type 3 Diabetes** – insulin resistance reaches the brain.
Even if the pancreas is working, neurons can't use
glucose properly, leading to memory and cognitive
problems.

IS IT THE PANCREAS OR THE INSULIN?

Here's the key:

- Sometimes, the pancreas **can't produce enough insulin**
(Type 1, late-stage Type 2).
- Other times, the pancreas is producing plenty, but the
cells refuse to listen (insulin resistance in Type 2).
- Often, it's a mix of both: the pancreas struggles more
and more over time because resistance makes the job
harder.

So the problem isn't always the pancreas itself—it's often the
way the body responds to insulin.

WHY THE PANCREAS GETS OVERWORKED

If you eat a lot of refined carbs and sugar, your pancreas has to
pump out insulin repeatedly, like an overworked employee
covering too many shifts. Over time, two things can happen:

1. **The cells stop responding.** They get "tired" of listening
to insulin's knock at the door and stop letting glucose in.
2. **The pancreas gets tired too.** It can't keep up with the
constant demand, so insulin production slows down.

This combination is what makes Type 2 diabetes progress.

THE HOPEFUL SIDE

Here's the good news: while you can't replace a failing pancreas, you *can* lighten its workload. Every time you balance your meals, move your body, reduce stress, or get enough sleep, you make the job easier. You give your pancreas space to do what it was designed to do.

Type 1, Type 2, Type 3—What's the Difference?

When I was first told I had diabetes, I thought there were only two kinds: the kind children get (Type 1) and the kind adults get (Type 2). It wasn't until much later that I learned there's more to the story. Understanding these types isn't just about medical definitions—it's about knowing how each one affects the body and, more importantly, the brain.

TYPE 1 DIABETES – WHEN THE PANCREAS STOPS WORKING

Type 1 diabetes is an **autoimmune disease.** The body's own immune system mistakenly attacks and destroys the insulin-producing cells in the pancreas. Without insulin, glucose can't enter the cells to be used for fuel.

- Usually begins in childhood or adolescence, but can appear at any age.
- Requires insulin injections for survival—there's no way around it.
- People with Type 1 must carefully balance food, activity, and insulin daily.

Think of Type 1 as a house without electricity—the fuel (glucose) is there, but without insulin, the lights can't turn on.

TYPE 2 DIABETES – WHEN THE CELLS STOP LISTENING

Type 2 diabetes, on the other hand, is mostly about **insulin resistance.** The pancreas is still making insulin—sometimes even too much—but the cells in the body stop responding. It's like someone constantly knocking at your door, and eventually, you stop answering.

- Usually develops in adulthood, but increasingly seen in children.
- Strongly linked to lifestyle factors: diet, inactivity, stress, weight, but also genetics.
- Often starts as **prediabetes**, with symptoms so subtle they go unnoticed for years.
- Medications like metformin or newer drugs can help, but lifestyle changes are powerful too.

In Type 2, the electricity works, but the appliances refuse to turn on—they're ignoring the signal.

TYPE 3 DIABETES – WHEN THE BRAIN GETS INVOLVED

Here's the type most people haven't heard of: **Type 3 Diabetes.**

This term is used by researchers to describe what happens when insulin resistance extends to the **brain.** Your neurons—your memory and thinking cells—need insulin to absorb glucose and function. When they can't, the brain begins to starve, even if the rest of the body has plenty of sugar in the blood.

- Strongly linked to Alzheimer's disease and other forms of dementia.
- Symptoms can start subtly: memory lapses, confusion, brain fog, mood swings, panic-like episodes.
- Over time, neurons shrink, connections weaken, and the brain loses its sharpness.

In Type 3, the lights flicker and fade—not because the house is out of power, but because the wiring has corroded.

WHY EVERY DIABETIC SHOULD CARE ABOUT THEIR BRAIN

Whether you have Type 1, Type 2, or even just prediabetes, here's the truth: your brain is always in the middle of the story.

- Blood sugar highs and lows directly affect mood, memory, and focus.
- Long-term instability increases the risk of dementia.
- Protecting your brain now means protecting your future independence, your relationships, and even your personality.

When I finally learned this, it hit me hard. Diabetes isn't just about avoiding complications "someday." It's about how you feel and function today—and how you safeguard your mind for tomorrow.

That's why this book is about more than balancing numbers. It's about keeping your brain, your memories, and your very self alive and well.

The Sugar–Brain Link: Alzheimer's, Dementia, and Type 3 Diabetes

A SILENT CONNECTION MOST PEOPLE MISS

When we think about diabetes, we picture the pancreas, blood sugar meters, and insulin injections. Rarely do we think about the brain. But in recent decades, scientists have uncovered something startling: unstable blood sugar and insulin resistance don't just strain the body — they can actually starve the brain. This discovery has led many researchers to call Alzheimer's disease *"Type 3 Diabetes."*

WHAT DEMENTIA REALLY IS

Dementia is not one single disease. It is a broad term describing a decline in memory, language, judgment, and daily functioning that is severe enough to interfere with normal life. While aging is a risk factor, dementia is not a "normal" part of growing older.

Symptoms often begin subtly: forgetting appointments, repeating questions, struggling to find words, or getting lost in familiar places. Over time, dementia robs people of their independence and sense of self.

ALZHEIMER'S DISEASE EXPLAINED

Alzheimer's is the most common form of dementia, accounting for about 60–80% of cases. In the Alzheimer's brain, several changes occur:

- **Amyloid plaques** – sticky protein clumps that build up between nerve cells, disrupting communication.
- **Tau tangles** – twisted protein fibers inside neurons that choke the cell from within.

- **Neuron death** – gradual destruction of brain cells, particularly in the hippocampus (the memory center).

As these changes progress, memory, reasoning, personality, and independence slip away.

WHY IT'S CALLED TYPE 3 DIABETES

Researchers began noticing that people with Type 2 diabetes had a much higher risk of developing Alzheimer's. But the connection went deeper than that.

- **Insulin resistance in the brain**: Just as muscles and fat cells can stop responding to insulin, so can neurons. This means the brain cannot properly absorb and use glucose — its main fuel.
- **Starved neurons**: When brain cells don't get enough energy, they misfire, leading to memory lapses, brain fog, mood swings, and eventually, cell death.
- **Sugar damage**: High blood sugar accelerates the formation of amyloid plaques and tau tangles, worsening the progression of Alzheimer's.
- **Inflammation and oxidative stress**: Chronic sugar spikes create inflammation that damages both blood vessels and brain tissue.

In short, Alzheimer's looks like the brain's version of diabetes — a condition where fuel is available, but the cells can't use it.

THE OVERLAP WITH BLOOD SUGAR SYMPTOMS

You may already recognize some of the early signs of brain glucose imbalance:

- Brain fog, word mix-ups, or difficulty focusing
- Vivid dreams or strange "night episodes"
- Mood swings or anxiety spikes after eating
- Forgetfulness that feels "too much for your age"
- A weird taste or sensation in the mouth when blood sugar is high

These are not just quirks of aging — they may be early red flags of the sugar–brain connection.

PROTECTING THE BRAIN THROUGH BLOOD SUGAR

The hopeful news is that the same strategies that balance blood sugar also protect the brain. You don't need futuristic medicine to start protecting your neurons today.

- **Balanced nutrition**: Eating protein, fiber, and healthy fats with carbs prevents sugar floods to the brain.
- **Movement**: A walk after meals lowers blood sugar and increases blood flow to the brain.
- **Stress reduction**: Cortisol spikes trigger sugar release. Meditation, Reiki, breathwork, or journaling calms the stress response.
- **Sleep**: Deep sleep activates the brain's glymphatic system — its "washing machine" that clears away amyloid plaques.
- **Herbs and spices**: Turmeric, rosemary, and sage are traditional brain tonics now backed by science. They reduce inflammation, support memory chemicals, and protect neurons.

Key Takeaway: Your Brain on Sugar

Alzheimer's and dementia are not random lightning strikes. In many cases, they are the long-term consequence of blood sugar imbalance and brain insulin resistance — what researchers now call **Type 3 Diabetes.**

This means you are not powerless. Every balanced meal, every walk, every night of good sleep, every mindful pause is not just protecting your pancreas — it is protecting your **memories, your clarity, and your future self.**

The sweetness of life does not come from sugar, but from a brain that stays sharp, connected, and present. By choosing balance today, you give your mind the gift of tomorrow.

Stress, Emotions & the Sugar–Brain Connection

1. STRESS HORMONES AND BLOOD SUGAR

When you experience stress — whether from an argument, financial worry, or even good excitement — your body flips into **"fight or flight" mode.**

- The adrenal glands release **cortisol** and **adrenaline.**
- These hormones tell the **liver** to dump stored glucose into the bloodstream.
- Why? Because in ancient times, stress meant danger, and your body needed instant fuel to fight or run.

The problem today is that stress rarely requires sprinting from a tiger. Instead, we sit at our desks or lie awake at night while glucose still surges — raising blood sugar without being burned off.

2. CHRONIC STRESS = CHRONIC HIGH SUGAR

When stress is occasional, the body bounces back. But **chronic stress** (bills, caregiving, deadlines, unresolved trauma) keeps cortisol elevated.

Effects:

- Blood sugar stays higher, even when eating well.
- Insulin resistance worsens (cells stop listening to insulin when cortisol is always around).
- Belly fat accumulates (cortisol signals fat storage in the abdomen).
- Sleep gets disrupted, fueling more sugar cravings.

3. STRESS & TYPE 1, TYPE 2, TYPE 3

- **Type 1 Diabetes:** Stress can worsen blood sugar fluctuations and increase the risk of dangerous highs and lows. Emotional stress may also trigger autoimmune flare-ups.
- **Type 2 Diabetes:** Stress is a major contributor to **insulin resistance.** Even without much sugar, chronic stress hormones can keep glucose elevated.
- **Type 3 Diabetes (Brain Insulin Resistance):** Chronic stress hormones inflame the brain, impair memory, and accelerate cognitive decline. Cortisol shrinks the hippocampus — the memory center of the brain.

4. STRESS, EMOTIONS & ALZHEIMER'S/DEMENTIA

Extreme or long-lasting stress doesn't just affect mood — it rewires the brain.

- **Cortisol damages neurons** in the hippocampus, making it harder to form or recall memories.
- **Inflammation spreads** throughout the brain, worsening insulin resistance.
- People with high lifetime stress levels show a higher risk of **Alzheimer's and other dementias.**
- Extreme emotions — grief, trauma, chronic anger, or anxiety — leave "imprints" on the nervous system that keep stress hormones cycling, even at rest.

5. HOW EXTREME EMOTIONS TRIGGER SUGAR & BRAIN IMBALANCE

- **Fear & panic:** Adrenaline floods → glucose spike → crash → shakiness, exhaustion.
- **Anger:** Raises blood pressure and cortisol → glucose rises.

- **Grief/sadness:** Often disrupts sleep and appetite, destabilizing sugar.
- **Excitement (even positive):** Still a stress state → can cause sugar rise in sensitive people.

In other words, it's not just diet — your **emotional climate** is constantly influencing your blood sugar and brain.

6. PROTECTION STRATEGIES: CALMING THE STRESS–SUGAR AXIS

Daily Nervous System Resets:

- **Breathing techniques** (box breathing, 4-7-8, alternate nostril) to lower cortisol.
- **Reiki or meditation** to shift from "fight or flight" into "rest and repair."
- **Journaling** to process emotions instead of holding them in the body.
- **Prayer or gratitude practice** → shown to reduce stress hormones and improve resilience.

Lifestyle Support:

- **Movement after stress:** Even a short walk burns off cortisol-driven glucose.
- **Good sleep hygiene:** Sleep is the body's reset button for stress and sugar.
- **Social connection:** Talking with friends, family, or support groups reduces stress hormones.

Nutritional Helpers:

- Magnesium-rich foods (leafy greens, nuts, seeds) calm nerves and muscles.
- Herbal teas: chamomile, lemon balm, holy basil (tulsi) reduce anxiety and stress-driven cravings.

- Adaptogens: ashwagandha, rhodiola — shown to reduce cortisol (use with guidance if on meds).

Key Takeaway

Stress is not just an emotion — it's a biochemical event that raises blood sugar, fuels insulin resistance, and accelerates brain decline. Extreme emotions — whether anger, grief, or panic — are real triggers that can tip your body into spikes and crashes.

By calming the stress–sugar axis daily, you protect both your **pancreas and your memory.** In the end, managing stress is not a luxury — it's medicine for your brain.

Part III – Natural Blood Sugar Balance

The Gut–Brain–Sugar Axis

YOUR GUT IS YOUR "SECOND BRAIN"

Inside your intestines live trillions of bacteria, viruses, and fungi collectively known as the **microbiome.** Far from being passive passengers, these microbes are busy chemists, producing neurotransmitters (brain chemicals), vitamins, and immune signals that shape your mood, cravings, and even blood sugar.

- **Serotonin (the "happiness" chemical):** ~90% is made in the gut.
- **Dopamine (the "motivation" chemical):** gut microbes help regulate its production.
- **GABA (the "calm" chemical):** produced in part by gut bacteria.

When your microbiome is balanced, your brain feels stable, focused, and energized. When it's out of balance, your mood, memory, and cravings suffer.

HOW BLOOD SUGAR AFFECTS THE MICROBIOME

- **High sugar intake** feeds harmful bacteria and yeast (like *Candida*). These microbes thrive on fast carbs and, in turn, send signals to your brain to **crave more sugar.**

- **Insulin resistance** often goes hand-in-hand with dysbiosis (imbalance between good and bad microbes).
- **Leaky gut**: high sugar and processed foods weaken the gut lining, letting inflammatory molecules leak into the bloodstream — worsening insulin resistance and brain inflammation.

This creates a vicious cycle:
Dysbiosis → cravings & brain fog → poor food choices → worse dysbiosis.

THE GUT–BRAIN–SUGAR CYCLE IN REAL LIFE

- Ever noticed sugar cravings right after you told yourself you'd "cut back"? That's your gut bugs screaming for their food source.
- Or felt brain fog and fatigue after processed carbs? That's inflammation signals traveling from the gut to the brain through the **vagus nerve.**

REBALANCING THE MICROBIOME FOR BLOOD SUGAR & BRAIN HEALTH
1. Probiotics (Good Bacteria)

- Found in fermented foods like yogurt, kefir, sauerkraut, kimchi, and miso.
- Supplements with strains like **Lactobacillus** and **Bifidobacterium** support insulin sensitivity and mood balance.

2. Prebiotics (Food for Good Bacteria)

- Fibers your body can't digest, but your microbes love.
- Found in garlic, onions, leeks, asparagus, artichokes, and oats.

- Feeding these fibers produces **short-chain fatty acids (SCFAs)** like butyrate, which reduce inflammation and improve blood sugar control.

3. Resistant Starch (The Special Carb)

- Unlike normal carbs, resistant starch resists digestion and feeds gut bacteria instead.
- Sources: cooled potatoes, green bananas, lentils, beans, oats.
- Benefits: improves insulin sensitivity, lowers post-meal glucose, feeds microbes that protect the brain.

WHY THIS MATTERS FOR TYPE 3 DIABETES

- A healthy microbiome = steady neurotransmitter production = clearer memory and mood.
- Dysbiosis = cravings, poor sleep, depression, and worsening insulin resistance.
- Gut health is directly tied to **Alzheimer's risk** — studies show people with dementia often have less microbial diversity and more "inflammatory" bacteria.

DAILY GUT–BRAIN RESET TIPS

1. **Eat fermented foods daily.** (Start with a spoonful, build up.)
2. **Add prebiotics at each meal.** (Onions, garlic, leafy greens, oats.)
3. **Use resistant starch smartly.** (Cook potatoes, then cool overnight and reheat — this lowers their glycemic impact.)
4. **Limit sugar and processed foods.** Starve the "bad bugs."
5. **Hydrate.** Water + herbal teas keep digestion smooth.

6. **Breathe.** The gut and brain talk via the vagus nerve — deep breathing and meditation strengthen this connection.

Key Takeaway: Your gut health shapes your brain health. By feeding the right microbes, you not only reduce cravings and balance blood sugar, but also protect your memory, mood, and long-term brain function. The gut–brain–sugar axis is the hidden key to preventing and managing Type 3 Diabetes.

Food as Medicine

THE BATTLE WITH CARB CRAVINGS

If there's one thing I know about blood sugar, it's that cravings can feel impossible to fight. For me, it takes about **three full days** to get over a craving—not just for sweets, but for any quick and easy *carb, like chips, crackers, etc..*

It wasn't always candy or dessert that pulled me in. Sometimes it was bread, pasta, crackers, or even something simple like toast. My body would act like it was starving, even when I had just finished eating. The feeling was so intense it was as if my body moved on autopilot, overriding my brain, pushing me to grab something—anything—that would quickly turn into sugar in my blood.

That's the grip carbs can have when blood sugar is unstable. It isn't just about willpower—it's body chemistry. Carbs break down quickly into glucose, and when your system has been trained to rely on that fast fuel, it sends out urgent survival signals until it gets the fix.

Here's the hopeful truth: if you can hold steady, the cravings fade. For me, by the third day, the noise quiets, the pull weakens, and I feel like myself again. That's when I remember—balance isn't about cutting out every carb forever. It's about learning which carbs work with your body, and how to pair them so they give you steady energy instead of rollercoaster crashes.

So how do we get there? It starts with building meals that bring the balance back.

PART 1 – THE FOUNDATIONS OF A BALANCED PLATE

Food is more than calories. It's information. Every bite you take tells your body what to do next—whether to release insulin in a rush, to stay steady, or to crash and burn. That's why one of the most powerful ways to balance blood sugar naturally is to learn how to build a meal that gives your body *stable energy* instead of sugar spikes and crashes.

THE THREE KEYS TO A BALANCED MEAL (THE "WHAT "ASPECT)

Think of your plate as a triangle. Each side represents one of the three macronutrients your body needs:

1. **Protein** – the anchor. Protein slows down digestion, prevents big spikes, and keeps you full longer.
   o Examples: eggs, chicken, turkey, fish, tofu, beans, lentils, Greek yogurt.
2. **Healthy Fats** – the stabilizer. Fat doesn't raise blood sugar at all, and when paired with carbs, it slows the release of glucose into the bloodstream.
   o Examples: avocado, nuts, seeds, olive oil, fatty fish, coconut.
3. **Fiber-rich Carbohydrates** – the gentle fuel. Not all carbs are the enemy—your brain needs glucose. The trick is choosing carbs that are high in fiber, which release sugar slowly.
   o Examples: leafy greens, colorful veggies, berries, apples, beans, lentils, quinoa, oats.

When all three are on your plate, your body gets steady energy without the rollercoaster.

What a Diabetic Body Needs:

Think of your plate as a triangle

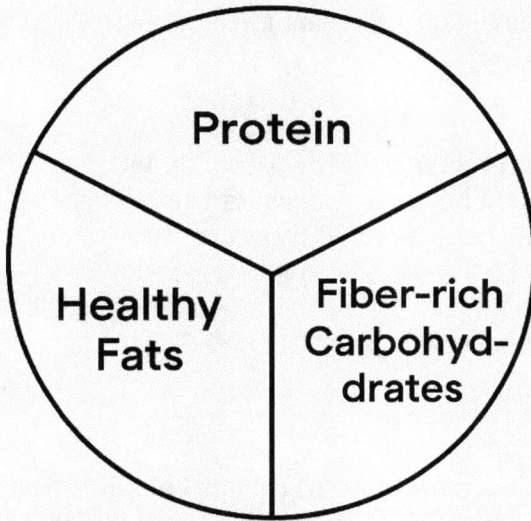

Protein

Healthy Fats

Fiber-rich Carbohyd-drates

THE 50/25/25 METHOD
(THE "HOW MUCH" ASPECT)

A simple way to remember balance is to divide your plate:

- **50% vegetables or salad** (fiber, vitamins, antioxidants).
- **25% protein** (to anchor the meal).
- **25% smart carbs** (whole grains, beans, starchy veggies) with a drizzle of healthy fat.

For example:

- Grilled salmon (protein + healthy fat)
- Steamed broccoli + mixed greens (fiber)
- Quinoa with olive oil (smart carb + fat)

This ratio isn't a diet—it's a framework for meals that keep you satisfied and balanced.

WHY THIS WORKS

When you eat carbs alone—like a bowl of white pasta or a muffin—your blood sugar spikes fast, then crashes hard. That's when you feel tired, shaky, or desperate for another snack.

But when you combine protein, fat, and fiber, the digestion process slows down. Glucose trickles into your blood instead of flooding it, giving your brain and body steady fuel.

It's like the difference between tossing paper on a fire (big flames, quick burnout) versus adding a log (slow, steady burn).

A PERSONAL EXAMPLE

When I was younger, lunch might be something quick like spaghetti or toast with jam. Within an hour, I'd be spacey, tired, or even acting like I was tipsy. That's because I was eating pure carbs, which sent my blood sugar soaring and then crashing.

Now, if I have spaghetti, I balance it. I'll choose whole-grain pasta, add a good portion of lean ground turkey or beans, load up on vegetables, and drizzle with olive oil. Same dish, completely different blood sugar response.

TWO SIMPLE VISUALS WORKING SIDE BY SIDE:

1. **The Triangle (Protein–Fat–Fiber)**
   - This is about the **components** of every meal.
   - It teaches: "Every plate needs these three building blocks."
   - Think of it like the *ingredients list* that keeps blood sugar steady.
2. **The 50/25/25 Plate Method**
   - This is about the **proportions** of food on your actual plate.
   - It teaches: "Here's how much of each food group should fill your plate."
   - Think of it like the *recipe directions* showing how to arrange the building blocks.

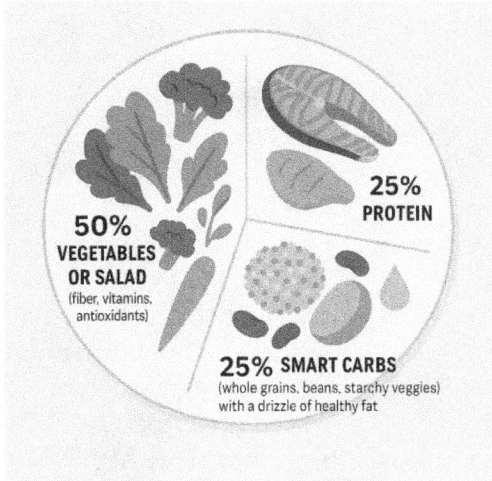

50%
VEGETABLES
OR SALAD
(fiber, vitamins,
antioxidants)

25%
PROTEIN

25% SMART CARBS
(whole grains, beans, starchy veggies)
with a drizzle of healthy fat

HOW THEY FIT TOGETHER

- **Protein side of the triangle** = your **25% protein on the plate**.
- **Healthy fat side of the triangle** = the drizzle or small portion that *complements* your plate (often combined with protein or smart carbs).
- **Fiber-rich carbs side of the triangle** = the **50% veggies/salad** + the **25% smart carbs** on the plate.

So:

- The **triangle** shows the *what* (all three must be present).
- The **50/25/25 plate** shows the *how much* (visual guide to proportions).

WHERE DO THE HEALTHY FATS COME IN?

Excellent question — because on the **50/25/25 plate visual**, it looks like fats are "missing." But actually, healthy fats are the **invisible glue** that weaves through the whole meal instead of taking up a section of the plate.

HERE'S HOW THEY FIT IN:
Where Healthy Fats Belong

- **With Protein**:
  - Salmon, eggs, nuts, or lean meats naturally contain healthy fats.
- **With Smart Carbs**:
  - Drizzle olive oil over quinoa, roast sweet potatoes in avocado oil, or sprinkle seeds on whole-grain toast.
- **With Vegetables (the big 50%)**:
  - Add olive oil to salad, avocado to greens, or sauté veggies in coconut oil.

WHY THEY'RE NOT A "SECTION" ON THE PLATE

Healthy fats don't need to be a large portion like protein or carbs. Instead, they're **paired with** or **cooked into** your protein, veggies, or carbs to slow digestion and stabilize blood sugar. Think of them as the **secret stabilizer** that turns a decent meal into a blood-sugar-friendly one.

So:

- The **triangle** diagram shows **protein, fat, and fiber carbs** as *must-have elements.*
- The **50/25/25 plate** shows **how much protein and carbs + veggies to aim for**, with **healthy fats worked in** across the plate.

PART 2 – FOODS THAT STABILIZE VS. FOODS THAT SPIKE

One of the most eye-opening lessons I've learned is that **not all carbs are created equal.** Some foods act like slow-burning logs on a fire, giving you steady warmth and energy. Others act like crumpled newspaper—quick flames, big smoke, and then nothing but ash.

When you start to notice the difference, it becomes much easier to choose foods that work with your body instead of against it.

FOODS THAT STABILIZE BLOOD SUGAR

These foods slow down digestion, prevent sugar spikes, and keep your energy steady:

- **Protein-Rich Foods**
  Eggs, fish, chicken, turkey, lean meats, tofu, tempeh, Greek yogurt, cottage cheese, beans, lentils.

- **Healthy Fats**
  Avocados, nuts, seeds, olive oil, coconut oil, fatty fish (salmon, mackerel, sardines), and nut butters.
- **Fiber-Rich Carbohydrates**
  Vegetables: leafy greens, broccoli, cauliflower, peppers, zucchini, carrots.
  Fruits: berries, apples, pears, citrus (lower sugar, high fiber).
  Whole Grains: quinoa, oats, barley, brown rice, buckwheat.
  Legumes: beans, chickpeas, lentils.
- **Herbs & Spices** (bonus stabilizers)
  Cinnamon, turmeric, ginger, and fenugreek — shown to improve insulin sensitivity.

These foods release glucose slowly, like a steady drip instead of a flood, giving your brain and body consistent fuel.

FOODS THAT SPIKE BLOOD SUGAR

These are the "quick-burning papers." They digest rapidly, flood your bloodstream with sugar, and often leave you crashing soon after.

- **Refined Carbohydrates**
  White bread, white rice, pasta made with white flour, crackers, bagels, and pastries.
- **Sugary Drinks & Foods**
  Soda, juice, sweetened coffee drinks, energy drinks, candy, desserts, and ice cream.
- **Processed Snacks**
  Chips, granola bars (many are loaded with hidden sugar), flavored yogurts, packaged breakfast cereals.
- **Alcohol**
  Especially mixed drinks with soda or juice. Alcohol also stresses the pancreas.

- **"Hidden Sugar" Foods**
  Ketchup, salad dressings, sauces, flavored coffees, even
  some health bars.

THE SURPRISE FOODS

Some foods seem healthy but can still spike blood sugar if eaten
alone:

- **Bananas, grapes, and tropical fruits** – better balanced
  with protein or fat (like nut butter).
- **Smoothies** – if mostly fruit, they hit like liquid sugar;
  better with protein powder or Greek yogurt.
- **"Whole wheat" bread** – many are still refined flours
  that act just like white bread.

A PERSONAL EXAMPLE

I remember grabbing a quick granola bar, thinking I was being
healthy. Within 30 minutes, I was shaky, irritable, and desperate
for another snack. Why? Because it was basically sugar
wrapped in oats.

Later, when I swapped that for an apple with almond butter, I
noticed a huge difference. The sweetness of the apple gave me
energy, but the fiber and fat kept me stable—same craving,
completely different outcome.

SIMPLE RULE OF THUMB

- **Stabilizers** = protein + fiber + healthy fat.
- **Spikers** = refined, processed, sugary, or carb-heavy
  foods eaten alone.

PROTEIN – THE ANCHOR

If blood sugar balance were a ship, protein would be the heavy anchor keeping it steady. Without enough protein, your meals act like waves tossing you around—up with a spike, down with a crash. With protein, digestion slows, glucose enters your bloodstream more gradually, and you stay fuller longer.

WHY PROTEIN MATTERS FOR BLOOD SUGAR

1. **Slows Digestion:** When protein is present in a meal, it delays how quickly carbohydrates are broken down into glucose. That means less of a sharp spike.
2. **Reduces Cravings:** Protein helps you feel satisfied, cutting down those "I need to eat something NOW" urges.
3. **Supports Muscle & Repair:** Muscles are big glucose burners. More lean muscle means better blood sugar control over time.
4. **Steadies Energy:** Protein gives your brain and body a steady trickle of fuel instead of a quick burst.

PROTEIN IN REAL LIFE MEALS

- **Breakfast:**
  Swap a plain bagel (spike city) for scrambled eggs with spinach. Or try Greek yogurt with berries and chia seeds.
- **Lunch:**
  Add grilled chicken or beans to your salad instead of just lettuce and dressing.
- **Snacks:**
  A boiled egg, turkey roll-ups, or a handful of roasted chickpeas keep you satisfied between meals.
- **Dinner:**
  Salmon with roasted veggies and quinoa steadies blood sugar far better than pasta with butter.

PROTEIN EXAMPLES BY CATEGORY

- **Animal-Based:**
  Eggs, chicken, turkey, fish (salmon, tuna, cod), beef
  (lean cuts), cottage cheese, Greek yogurt.
- **Plant-Based:**
  Tofu, tempeh, beans (black beans, kidney beans, pinto
  beans), lentils, chickpeas, edamame, quinoa.
- **Snackable Proteins:**
  Nuts, seeds, protein smoothies (without added sugar),
  roasted chickpeas.

A PERSONAL REFLECTION

Looking back, I can see the difference when protein was
missing. A lunch of spaghetti left me foggy and spacey. But
when I added lean turkey or beans into the same dish, it felt
completely different—no dizzy "high," no crash, no wandering
brain. Just steady energy.

HEALTHY FATS – THE STABILIZER

If protein is the anchor that steadies the ship, then healthy fats
are the ballast that keeps you from tipping over. Fats don't raise
blood sugar at all. Instead, when paired with carbohydrates,
they *slow the release of glucose* into the bloodstream,
preventing those sharp rises and sudden crashes.

WHY HEALTHY FATS MATTER FOR BLOOD SUGAR

1. **Zero Spike:** Unlike carbs, fats don't convert to sugar, so
   they have no direct impact on blood glucose levels.
2. **Slower Digestion:** When you pair fat with carbs, it
   slows stomach emptying, releasing glucose at a steady
   trickle instead of a flood.

3. **Brain Fuel:** Your brain is made of nearly 60% fat. Healthy fats keep it sharp, improving focus, memory, and mood.
4. **Hormone Balance:** Insulin is a hormone—and so are the ones that regulate hunger and energy. Healthy fats help stabilize them.

HEALTHY FATS IN REAL LIFE MEALS

- **Breakfast:**
  Add avocado slices to eggs, or sprinkle chia seeds on Greek yogurt.
- **Lunch:**
  Top your salad with olive oil and pumpkin seeds instead of a sugary dressing.
- **Snacks:**
  A small handful of almonds, walnuts, or sunflower seeds can stop a mid-afternoon crash.
- **Dinner:**
  Grill salmon (rich in omega-3s) or drizzle olive oil over roasted veggies.

EXAMPLES OF HEALTHY FATS

- **Plant-Based Fats:**
  Avocados, olives, olive oil, nuts (almonds, walnuts, cashews), seeds (chia, flax, pumpkin, sunflower), coconut, and coconut oil.
- **Animal-Based Fats:**
  Fatty fish (salmon, sardines, mackerel, trout), pasture-raised eggs, grass-fed butter (in moderation).
- **Hidden Add-Ins:**
  Nut butters (almond, peanut, cashew) — great paired with fruit for blood sugar balance.

A PERSONAL REFLECTION

For years, I was taught to avoid fat—"low-fat" this, "fat-free" that. But I noticed something: those "fat-free" foods always made me hungrier later, and my brain felt foggy. When I added healthy fats back in—avocado on toast, olive oil on salads, salmon for dinner—my energy lasted longer, my mind felt clearer, and the desperate carb cravings started to calm down.

FIBER-RICH CARBOHYDRATES – THE GENTLE FUEL

Carbohydrates often get a bad reputation, but the truth is, your brain *needs* glucose to function. The problem isn't carbs themselves—it's the kind of carbs you choose. The right ones act like **gentle, slow-burning fuel**; the wrong ones act like lighter fluid, flaring up fast and burning out just as quickly.

WHY FIBER MATTERS FOR BLOOD SUGAR

1. **Slows Sugar Release:** Fiber acts like a traffic cop, controlling how quickly glucose enters the bloodstream.
2. **Feeds Your Gut:** Fiber nourishes healthy gut bacteria, which in turn improves insulin sensitivity.
3. **Steady Energy:** Fiber-rich carbs give your brain and body a gradual, sustainable flow of glucose.
4. **Craving Control:** The more fiber in your meal, the less likely you are to crave sugar later.

COMPLEX VS. SIMPLE CARBS

- **Simple Carbohydrates**
  - Found in foods like white bread, pastries, soda, candy, and fruit juice.
  - Made of short sugar chains that digest rapidly, causing sharp spikes and quick crashes.
  - Think: instant energy, but gone in a flash.
- **Complex Carbohydrates**

- o Found in whole grains, beans, lentils, vegetables, and fruits with skins.
- o Packed with fiber, vitamins, and minerals.
- o Digest slowly, releasing glucose steadily—fuel that lasts.
- o Think: slow-burning logs on a fire, not paper that flames up and disappears.

FIBER-RICH CARBS IN REAL LIFE MEALS

- **Breakfast:**
  Swap sugary cereal for steel-cut oats with berries and chia seeds.
- **Lunch:**
  Pair quinoa or lentils with roasted veggies for a nourishing grain bowl.
- **Snacks:**
  An apple with the skin + a handful of nuts beats crackers or granola bars any day.
- **Dinner:**
  A plate with half non-starchy veggies (broccoli, peppers, spinach) alongside a smaller portion of sweet potato or brown rice.

EXAMPLES OF FIBER-RICH CARBOHYDRATES

- **Vegetables:** Leafy greens, broccoli, carrots, peppers, zucchini, cauliflower.
- **Fruits:** Berries, apples, pears, citrus (fiber-rich and lower sugar).
- **Whole Grains:** Quinoa, oats, barley, brown rice, buckwheat.
- **Legumes:** Lentils, beans, chickpeas.
- **Starchy Veggies (in moderation):** Sweet potatoes, squash, beets.

A PERSONAL REFLECTION

For years, I lumped all carbs together as "bad." But I started noticing something: pasta left me foggy, hungry, and irritable an hour later, while a quinoa salad with beans and veggies gave me steady energy all afternoon. Once I understood that the difference was **fiber**, it finally made sense. My body didn't hate carbs—it hated the fast-burning ones.

SUPPLEMENTS & HERBS – HELPERS WITH CAUTION

Food is the foundation for balancing blood sugar, but certain supplements and herbs can offer additional support. The key is understanding that while many are natural, they are also *powerful*—and if you're already on medication, combining the two could lead to blood sugar dropping too low (hypoglycemia) or other side effects. Always check with a healthcare professional before starting anything new.

SUPPLEMENTS THAT MAY SUPPORT BLOOD SUGAR

- **Magnesium** – Many people with diabetes are low in magnesium. It helps the body use insulin more effectively and may reduce insulin resistance.
- **Chromium** – Plays a role in carb and fat metabolism; may improve insulin sensitivity.
- **Alpha-Lipoic Acid (ALA)** – An antioxidant that supports nerve health and may improve insulin sensitivity.
- **Vitamin D** – Deficiency is linked with insulin resistance and a higher risk of diabetes.
- **Omega-3 Fatty Acids (Fish Oil or Algal Oil)** – Help reduce inflammation and support heart health, which is extra important for people with diabetes.

HERBS TRADITIONALLY USED FOR BLOOD SUGAR SUPPORT

- **Cinnamon** – May help improve insulin sensitivity and lower fasting blood sugar.
- **Fenugreek** – Seeds are high in soluble fiber and may help slow digestion and sugar absorption.
- **Bitter Melon** – Used in traditional medicine; may act like natural insulin.
- **Gymnema Sylvestre** – Nicknamed the "sugar destroyer" because it can reduce sugar absorption and cravings.
- **Turmeric (Curcumin)** – Anti-inflammatory and may support insulin sensitivity.

IMPORTANT CAUTIONS

Because supplements and herbs can **amplify the effect of diabetes medications**, they can sometimes push blood sugar **too low.** This is especially important if you are on:

- **Metformin** (can interact with herbs that lower sugar too strongly).
- **Sulfonylureas** (like glipizide, glyburide, etc., which increase insulin release).
- **Insulin injections** (highest risk of hypoglycemia when combined with sugar-lowering herbs).
- **SGLT2 inhibitors** (like Jardiance/empagliflozin – could interact with diuretics and herbs affecting the kidneys).

A PRACTICAL APPROACH

1. **Start with food first.** No supplement can outdo an unbalanced diet.
2. **Add one thing at a time.** If you decide to try a supplement or herb, track your blood sugar closely.
3. **Check interactions, e**specially if you're on prescription meds.
4. **Think "support," not "magic pill."** Herbs and supplements work best when layered onto a foundation of balanced meals, movement, stress management, and sleep.

PERSONAL REFLECTION

When I first started learning about natural options, I wanted to try everything. Cinnamon in my tea, turmeric in my food, bottles of supplements on my shelf. But I quickly learned that my blood sugar could dip too low if I wasn't careful. What helped most was focusing on **one supportive change at a time**—and letting food be the first medicine.

FOODS & HERBS THAT SUPPORT THE PANCREAS

While there's no magic cure for pancreatic health, certain foods and herbs can **reduce inflammation, improve insulin sensitivity, and ease stress on the pancreas.** Think of them as gentle allies, not quick fixes.

BITTER FOODS

Arugula, dandelion greens, kale, and mustard greens — bitter flavors stimulate digestion and encourage healthy pancreatic enzyme flow.

ANTIOXIDANT-RICH FRUITS

Blueberries and cherries are loaded with antioxidants that help reduce oxidative stress and protect delicate pancreatic tissue.

CRUCIFEROUS VEGETABLES

Broccoli, Brussels sprouts, and cauliflower support detox pathways and lower inflammation throughout the body.

ANTI-INFLAMMATORY SPICES

- **Turmeric:** Research suggests curcumin may help protect pancreatic cells from damage.
- **Ginger:** Improves digestion and calms inflammation.
- **Cinnamon:** Helps regulate blood sugar by improving insulin sensitivity.
- **Fenugreek seeds:** Used for centuries in traditional medicine to lower blood sugar and protect pancreatic function.

SULFUR-RICH FOODS

Garlic and onions offer anti-inflammatory compounds and may also enhance insulin sensitivity.

GREEN TEA

Rich in catechins, which fight both inflammation and oxidative stress.

TEAS FOR PANCREATIC & BLOOD SUGAR SUPPORT

A warm cup of tea can be a simple way to incorporate healing herbs:

- **Dandelion root tea** – gently bitter, supporting both the liver and pancreas.
- **Turmeric + ginger tea** – a soothing anti-inflammatory blend.
- **Cinnamon tea** – helps stabilize blood sugar and curb cravings.
- **Fenugreek tea** – a traditional remedy for blood sugar regulation.

LIFESTYLE SUPPORT – A GENTLE "CLEANSE" FOR THE PANCREAS

Forget harsh detoxes—the best way to support your pancreas is to **reduce its workload**:

1. **Cut refined sugar & processed carbs** → fewer insulin spikes means less stress.
2. **Build balanced meals** (protein + fiber + healthy fat with carbs) → steadier energy.
3. **Stay hydrated** → water supports digestion and circulation.
4. **Avoid overeating** → smaller meals ease the demand on insulin and enzymes.
5. **Limit alcohol** → alcohol heavily burdens the pancreas and can trigger inflammation.
6. **Gentle fasting or meal spacing** (if safe for you) → gives the pancreas rest periods.
7. **Daily movement** → exercise reduces insulin resistance, so the pancreas doesn't have to work as hard.

IMPORTANT NOTE

There's no "reset button" or miracle herb for the pancreas. But with consistent care—anti-inflammatory foods, herbal teas, balanced meals, and mindful lifestyle habits—you can **lighten the pancreas' load, improve insulin sensitivity, and slow the progression of insulin resistance.**

The Order of Eating for Blood Sugar Balance

1. VEGGIES FIRST (FIBER)

- Non-starchy vegetables (like salad, broccoli, spinach, zucchini) create a "fiber shield" in your gut.
- Fiber slows the breakdown of carbs and delays glucose absorption.
- Example: Start with a salad or steamed veggies.

2. PROTEIN & HEALTHY FATS

- Protein (chicken, fish, eggs, beans) and fats (olive oil, avocado, nuts) further slow digestion.
- They "anchor" the meal, keeping blood sugar steady.
- Example: After your salad, eat your grilled chicken or salmon.

3. SMART CARBS LAST

- Whole grains, beans, lentils, sweet potatoes, or fruit should come at the end.
- Eating carbs last means your blood sugar rise is gentler, because the fiber + protein + fat buffer is already in place.
- Example: Finish with quinoa, beans, or a small serving of sweet potato.

WHY THIS WORKS

- When carbs go in first → **fast spike.**
- When carbs go in last → **slow, controlled rise.**
- This reduces insulin demand, keeps you fuller longer, and minimizes cravings later.

PRACTICAL TIPS FOR FOOD ORDER

- **At restaurants:** Eat the side salad first, then protein, then carbs.
- **At home:** Build your plate but eat in the 1-2-3 sequence (veggies → protein/fat → carbs).
- **Snacking hack:** If you want fruit, pair it with nuts or cheese, not by itself.

BY DIABETES TYPE

- **Type 1:** Still must dose insulin, but food order can reduce extreme highs/lows.
- **Type 2:** Very effective — studies show a **40% lower post-meal glucose** when following a food order.
- **Type 3:** Especially helpful for brain health — prevents the sugar flood that triggers brain fog, cravings, or nighttime episodes.

Key Takeaway: What goes into your mouth *first* matters. **Veggies → protein/fat → carbs** is the order that keeps blood sugar most stable.

FOOD ORDER WHEN FOODS ARE MIXED
1. The Science of Order Still Applies

Even when foods are eaten together, your digestive system processes them in the **same order**:

- **Fiber** (veggies, legumes, nuts, seeds) forms a gel-like barrier in the stomach and small intestine. This slows down carb absorption.
- **Protein and fats** take longer to digest → they keep food in the stomach longer.
- **Carbs** (especially simple carbs) are digested fastest. If eaten alone, they rush into the bloodstream. But if "trapped" in fiber and fat, their release slows.

2. What Happens in a Mixed Meal

Imagine a plate of salmon, broccoli, and rice eaten together:

- The **fiber in broccoli** mixes with rice, slowing its breakdown.
- The **protein and fat in salmon** slow stomach emptying, so the rice trickles out gradually.
- Result: a smoother glucose curve compared to eating rice alone.

Now imagine rice eaten alone: it shoots into the bloodstream fast → spike → crash.

3. Practical Eating Tips (Even with Mixed Meals)

- **Bites matter.** If you take a forkful that's mostly rice or bread, you're still getting a faster hit of carbs. If you combine bites (protein + veg + carb), digestion is more balanced.
- **Chewing matters.** Chew thoroughly (20–30 chews), especially carbs → this slows down how quickly glucose is available.
- **Small portions of carbs.** If the carb portion is smaller (25% of the plate), its effect is muted by protein/fiber.

4. Real-Life Scenarios

- **Sandwich:** White bread alone = sugar rush. Sandwich with turkey, cheese, lettuce, and avocado = slower digestion (protein + fat + fiber buffer).
- **Pasta:** Plain spaghetti = spike. Pasta with chicken + spinach + olive oil = slower release.
- **Smoothies:** Fruit-only smoothie = naked carbs. Add Greek yogurt, chia seeds, or nut butter = balanced.

5. Best Rule of Thumb for Mixed Meals

Always make sure protein and/or fiber are present with carbs.

Even if you're eating them in the same bite, your body sorts them out in the right order:

- Fiber forms a protective shield.
- Protein/fats anchor digestion.
- Carbs are slowed down and released more gently.

Key Takeaway:
In mixed meals, food order still influences digestion, but **composition matters more**. As long as your plate follows the **50/25/25 rule (veggies/protein/carbs + fat)**, you don't have to stress about separating foods. What matters is that every carb is "dressed" with fiber, protein, or fat.

The Journey of Food: Why Order & Chewing Matter

1. CHEWING & SALIVA – DIGESTION STARTS IN THE MOUTH

Mechanical Breakdown

- When you chew, your teeth grind food into smaller pieces, increasing the surface area.
- The more finely food is broken down, the easier it is for enzymes and stomach acid to do their job later.
- Poorly chewed food → larger chunks → harder to digest → faster glucose release once it hits the small intestine (because the carbs aren't "buffered" properly).

Saliva: Your First Digestive Fluid

- Saliva is 98% water, but the other 2% contains enzymes, electrolytes, and antimicrobial compounds.
- The key enzyme for blood sugar is **salivary amylase**, which immediately starts breaking down starches (bread, rice, pasta, potatoes) into smaller sugar molecules (maltose, dextrins).
- That means the digestion of carbs **literally starts before you swallow.**
- Fun fact: if you hold a cracker in your mouth long enough without chewing, it will start tasting sweet — that's amylase in action.

Why Chewing Slows Blood Sugar Release

- If you chew thoroughly, the food mixes evenly with saliva.
- This coats carbs in enzymes while also pacing how fast you swallow → slower stomach emptying later.

- If you eat too quickly, carbs enter your stomach in larger pieces, bypassing saliva's full effect. This often leads to a **bigger, faster glucose dump** in the small intestine.

Nervous System Connection: The Cephalic Phase

- Chewing and tasting also trigger your nervous system to **"prepare the body"**: stomach acid increases, pancreatic enzymes begin preparing, and insulin secretion may even start in anticipation.
- Eating too fast or not chewing enough can confuse this process — your brain doesn't have time to send the right signals, leading to digestion problems and erratic blood sugar.

Chewing & Hormone Release

- Slow chewing helps release hormones like **GLP-1** and **CCK** from the gut, which:
  - Tell the brain, "I'm getting full."
  - Slow stomach emptying → steadier glucose release.
- If you rush your meal, these hormones don't get time to activate, and you may overeat without realizing it.

Practical Tips

- **Aim for 20–30 chews per bite**, especially for starchy carbs (bread, rice, potatoes).
- **Put your fork down** between bites to naturally slow the pace.
- **Notice sweetness:** With enough chewing, you'll taste natural sugars emerging in foods like grains, carrots, or even nuts.
- **Mindful eating:** Paying attention to texture and flavor helps regulate both digestion and portion size.

Key Takeaway: Chewing isn't just about breaking down food — it's the first lever for controlling blood sugar. The slower and more thorough you chew, the smoother your glucose enters your bloodstream, the calmer your pancreas works, and the fewer cravings you face later.

CHEWING, DENTAL HEALTH & BLOOD SUGAR BALANCE

1. Teeth: The First Grinders

- Your teeth are like the "blades of a food processor." If they're strong and aligned, they grind food into small, even particles.
- Missing teeth, dental pain, or ill-fitting dentures result in larger chunks of food being swallowed, less saliva mixing, and a faster rise in blood sugar later.
- People with poor dental health may unconsciously **avoid fibrous foods** (like raw veggies, nuts, seeds) and lean toward soft, processed carbs — which spike blood sugar faster.

2. TMJ (Temporomandibular Joint Disorder)

- TMJ can cause pain, stiffness, or fatigue when chewing.
- This often leads to **minimal chewing** (swallowing food more quickly or in larger pieces).
- Larger pieces of starchy food = less pre-digestion in the mouth = a **quicker, harsher blood sugar spike** in the intestine.
- People with TMJ may prefer soft foods — which tend to be carb-heavy (mashed potatoes, pasta, bread) unless they're consciously choosing high-protein or blended veggie options.

3. Saliva & Dental Health

- Healthy saliva flow is vital for:
  - o Washing away bacteria
  - o Beginning carb digestion (amylase)
  - o Neutralizing acids
- **Dry mouth (xerostomia)** — often caused by medications, age, or dehydration — reduces enzyme activity and makes swallowing harder. This can push people toward liquid carbs (juices, sodas, smoothies) that flood the bloodstream quickly.

4. Dental Infections & Inflammation

- Gum disease (periodontitis) isn't just a mouth problem — it's linked to **systemic inflammation** and **higher insulin resistance.**
- Chronic gum inflammation can worsen blood sugar control, creating a vicious cycle (high blood sugar → gum disease risk → gum disease → worse blood sugar).

Practical Solutions if Chewing Is Hard

1. **Blended & Pureed Foods (but balanced):**
   - o Smoothies with **protein + veggies + healthy fats** (not fruit-only sugar bombs).
   - o Pureed soups (lentils, beans, spinach, cauliflower).
2. **Soft Yet Protein-Rich Options:**
   - o Scrambled eggs, Greek yogurt, cottage cheese.
   - o Steamed fish or tender chicken.
   - o Well-cooked beans and lentils.
3. **Chew-Friendly Veggies:**
   - o Steamed zucchini, spinach, mushrooms.
   - o Mashed cauliflower instead of mashed potatoes.
4. **Dental Care & Support:**
   - o Hydrate for saliva flow.

- o Sugar-free gum (with xylitol) stimulates saliva + helps protect teeth.
- o Regular dental check-ups (gum health directly impacts blood sugar).

Key Takeaway: If you struggle with chewing (TMJ, dentures, missing teeth, dry mouth), you're at higher risk of favoring **soft, high-carb foods** that spike blood sugar. The key is to adapt with **soft but balanced foods** (protein + veggies + fats) and take extra care of dental health, since gum inflammation itself worsens insulin resistance.

2. STOMACH – MIXING & SLOW RELEASE
The Churning Chamber

- After chewing and swallowing, food enters the stomach, where it's churned into a semi-liquid mixture called **chyme**.
- Stomach acid (hydrochloric acid) + digestive enzymes (like pepsin for protein) begin breaking food into smaller molecules.
- This isn't just about digestion — the stomach also **controls timing**: how quickly food leaves and enters the small intestine (where glucose absorption happens).

Protein & Fat: The Slow-Digesters

- **Protein** (eggs, meat, fish, tofu, beans) takes longer to break down, so it delays stomach emptying.
- **Fat** (avocado, olive oil, nuts, fish) is even slower to digest, sending a message to the stomach to "hold onto food longer."
- Together, protein and fat act like a **traffic light** at the stomach's exit: they slow down how fast carbs move forward, which prevents glucose from flooding the bloodstream all at once.

Fiber: The Gel-Forming Shield

- **Soluble fiber** (found in veggies, beans, oats, flax, apples) absorbs water and forms a gel in the stomach.
- This gel literally coats the meal, making it harder for digestive enzymes to reach carbs.
- Result: Glucose is "drip-fed" into the bloodstream instead of dumped.
- **Insoluble fiber** (leafy greens, broccoli, nuts, seeds) doesn't gel as much, but it adds *bulk* and helps regulate stomach emptying too.

Why Food Order Matters in the Stomach

- If you eat **veggies first** → fiber coats the stomach lining, creating the gel barrier.
- If you eat **protein and fat next** → the stomach holds the food longer, mixing everything slowly.
- If you eat **carbs last** → by the time they enter the small intestine, they're slowed by both the fiber barrier and the protein/fat delay.
- If you eat **carbs first** → they slip through quickly, hit the small intestine unprotected, and spike blood sugar.

Hormonal Signals From the Stomach

- The stomach also communicates with your brain and pancreas:
  - **Ghrelin (hunger hormone):** Drops once the stomach stretches and protein is detected.
  - **GLP-1 and CCK (fullness hormones):** Triggered by fat and protein, telling your brain you're satisfied.
  - These hormones slow stomach emptying further, giving your body time to process nutrients.

Practical Tips for Using the Stomach's Power

1. **Eat in order:** Veggies → protein/fat → carbs.
2. **Add fiber to every meal:** Even 1 cup of leafy greens or ½ cup of beans makes a difference.
3. **Include some fat:** A drizzle of olive oil, avocado, or a handful of nuts slows stomach emptying and prolongs satiety.
4. **Don't rush eating:** Stomach-brain signaling (fullness) takes ~20 minutes. Eating too fast bypasses your natural stop signs.

Key Takeaway: The stomach isn't just a container — it's a smart traffic controller. Protein, fat, and fiber tell it to **slow down**, while carbs alone rush through. By eating in the right order, you train your stomach to drip-feed glucose into your bloodstream — keeping your energy steady, your pancreas calmer, and your brain clearer.

3. SMALL INTESTINE – THE GATEWAY TO THE BLOODSTREAM
The Workhorse of Digestion

- The **small intestine** (about 20 feet long!) is where **90% of nutrient absorption** takes place.
- By the time food reaches here, the stomach has liquefied it into **chyme** (a semi-digested soup).
- Now, specialized enzymes finish the job of breaking down proteins, fats, and especially **carbohydrates**.

Carbohydrate Breakdown → Glucose

- Enzymes from the pancreas (like **amylase, maltase, sucrase, and lactase**) chop carbs into **single sugar molecules** (mainly glucose).
- These molecules pass through the intestinal lining and enter the bloodstream.

- **How fast this happens depends on what came before it:**
  - o **Fiber-first meal:** Fiber forms a barrier, so glucose trickles out slowly.
  - o **Protein/fat-rich meal:** Slows stomach emptying → smaller, steadier glucose release.
  - o **Carbs-first meal:** No protection → glucose pours into the bloodstream, spiking sugar.

The Bloodstream Connection

- Once glucose enters the blood, your **pancreas** releases insulin to move it into cells (muscle, liver, fat).
- **Steady trickle = gentle insulin response.**
- **Sugar flood = insulin surge**, followed by a crash that triggers cravings, fatigue, or shakiness.

The Gut–Brain Axis

- The small intestine doesn't just digest — it talks to your brain via hormones and nerves.
- **Incretins (GLP-1, GIP):** Released here when nutrients are detected.
  - o They signal the pancreas to release insulin.
  - o They also slow down digestion to prevent overload.
- If meals are balanced, incretins keep things calm. If meals are carb-heavy, they get overwhelmed.

The Role of the Microbiome

- The lower small intestine houses part of your **gut microbiome**.
- Good bacteria feed on fiber and resistant starch, producing **short-chain fatty acids (SCFAs)** that improve insulin sensitivity.

- Bad bacteria thrive on sugar → inflammation → worsened insulin resistance and cravings.
- This is why fiber and plant foods are so protective against diabetes progression.

If You Ate Veggies + Protein/Fat First...

☑ Glucose enters bloodstream slowly.
☑ Pancreas doesn't overwork.
☑ Energy feels steady, cravings are weaker.
☑ Brain receives consistent fuel → less fog, better memory.

If You Ate Carbs First...

✖ Glucose floods the blood.
✖ Pancreas pumps out a surge of insulin.
✖ Crash follows, with shakiness, hunger, and irritability.
✖ Brain gets hit with a "sugar wave" then a drought, worsening memory and mood swings.

Practical Tips for Small Intestine Balance

1. **Eat carbs last** → protect the bloodstream from a flood.
2. **Always pair carbs with protein/fat** → never naked carbs.
3. **Feed your microbiome** → daily fiber, beans, veggies, fermented foods (sauerkraut, kefir, kimchi).
4. **Chew thoroughly** → digestion that starts early is easier to regulate downstream.

Key Takeaway: The small intestine is the **gateway to your bloodstream.** Every bite of carbs eventually becomes glucose here — but *how fast and how much* depends entirely on what you ate with it. Veggies, protein, and fat act like gatekeepers, turning sugar floods into steady streams.

4. BLOODSTREAM – ENERGY & INSULIN RESPONSE
Glucose Enters the Blood

- Once carbs are fully digested in the small intestine, glucose molecules pass through the gut wall into the bloodstream.
- This raises **blood sugar (blood glucose levels).**
- The body *wants balance* — not too high, not too low — so it calls on the **pancreas** to help.

The Role of Insulin

- The pancreas releases **insulin**, a hormone that works like a "key."
- Insulin unlocks cells (muscle, liver, fat) so glucose can move inside and be used for **energy** or stored for later.
- **Muscle cells:** burn glucose for movement.
- **Liver cells:** store glucose as glycogen.
- **Fat cells:** store extra glucose as body fat when storage is full.

Slow Entry = Smooth Ride

- If glucose enters slowly (because you ate veggies first, protein/fat with carbs, and chewed thoroughly):
  - ☑ Insulin rises gently.
  - ☑ Glucose slips into cells without drama.
  - ☑ Blood sugar stays steady → energy feels even, mood stable, brain clear.
- This is the **ideal state** — steady energy, no rollercoaster.

Fast Entry = Sugar Rollercoaster

- If glucose floods in quickly (from soda, bread, white rice, pasta, sweets):
  - ✗ Insulin surges high to force sugar into cells.
  - ✗ Blood sugar plummets after (the "crash").

✖ Crash symptoms: shakiness, urgent hunger, irritability, fatigue, brain fog.

✖ Brain misreads this as "danger" and demands **more carbs → cravings.**

- This is the vicious cycle many people live in daily.

Insulin Resistance & the Bloodstream

- Over time, if the body is constantly bombarded with glucose surges:
  o Cells stop responding well to insulin.
  o The pancreas has to pump out *more and more insulin.*
  o Blood sugar stays high anyway → **insulin resistance.**
- This is the root problem in **Type 2 diabetes and Type 3 (brain insulin resistance).**

Brain & Blood Sugar

- The brain is a "sugar hog" — it uses about **20% of all glucose energy.**
- But it hates swings. Spikes followed by crashes confuse memory, focus, and mood.
- Smooth glucose entry = sharp thinking, stable emotions.
- Chaotic glucose entry = brain fog, irritability, word mix-ups, vivid dream "episodes."

Practical Ways to Smooth Bloodstream Entry

1. **Food order:** Veggies → protein/fat → carbs.
2. **Balanced plates:** 50/25/25 (half veggies, quarter protein, quarter smart carbs with fat).
3. **Move after meals:** Walking helps muscles pull glucose from blood (lowers spikes).
4. **Stress control:** Cortisol pushes extra glucose into the blood even without food.

5. **Avoid naked carbs:** Always pair carbs with protein/fat.

Key Takeaway: The bloodstream is the **bridge** between what you eat and how you feel. Every spike and crash is your body's way of saying, *"Balance me."* Smooth entry means steady energy, a calm brain, and protection against long-term insulin resistance.

5. LARGE INTESTINE & BOWELS – THE FINAL PHASE
Fiber Feeds the Gut

- Not all carbs are digested in the small intestine.
- **Soluble fiber** (beans, oats, apples, flax) travels into the large intestine, where it becomes food for gut bacteria.
- Good bacteria ferment this fiber into **short-chain fatty acids (SCFAs)** like butyrate, acetate, and propionate.
- These compounds:
  - ☑ Improve **insulin sensitivity** (cells use sugar better).
  - ☑ Reduce **inflammation** (critical in diabetes prevention).
  - ☑ Influence **hunger hormones** (like ghrelin and GLP-1), helping regulate appetite.

The Microbiome–Brain Connection (The Gut–Brain Axis)

- Your intestines and brain talk constantly through the **vagus nerve** and chemical messengers.
- Microbes in your colon produce neurotransmitters like **serotonin, dopamine, and GABA** — all of which affect mood, sleep, memory, and even dreams.
- Imbalances (too much sugar, too few fibers) → microbial shifts that worsen cravings, anxiety, brain fog.
- A balanced microbiome = steadier blood sugar *and* steadier thoughts.

Bowel Movements as a Blood Sugar Signal

- Regular bowel movements show that fiber is doing its job, sweeping out waste and excess hormones.
- Constipation can worsen insulin resistance and make blood sugar harder to control.
- Loose stools can mean poor absorption of nutrients that stabilize blood sugar.

My Observation: Dreams, Memory, and Weird Tastes Before a Bowel Movement

This is actually very insightful. What may be happening:

1. **Neurochemical surge:** Right before a bowel movement, the gut releases signaling molecules that interact with the brain (serotonin, especially — ~90% of serotonin is made in the gut). This can trigger vivid dreams, flashes of memory, or even "phantom tastes."
2. **Blood sugar shift:** Digestion slows while the body prepares for elimination, sometimes triggering a brief **drop in blood sugar** → leading to sensations like brain fog, panic, or odd sensory input.
3. **Vagus nerve stimulation:** The act of moving the bowels stimulates the vagus nerve, which connects directly to brain centers for memory, mood, and autonomic function. That's why people sometimes feel lightheaded, flushed, or emotional before/during elimination.
4. **Toxin signaling:** If waste has been sitting in the colon, certain byproducts (like ammonia or short-chain amines) may briefly affect brain function before release — potentially triggering those strange "memory-taste-dream" episodes I've described.

Practical Tips for Large Intestine Health

1. **Feed your microbiome daily:** beans, lentils, leafy greens, onions, garlic, fermented foods.
2. **Hydrate:** water keeps stools moving and prevents "toxic backlog."
3. **Support elimination timing:** a regular schedule reduces the build-up of signals that may affect brain and memory.
4. **Move after meals:** light walking massages the intestines and helps regularity.
5. **Notice patterns:** If dreams/memory/taste episodes always precede bowel movements, track what foods make them stronger or weaker — this may reveal food sensitivities or microbial shifts.

Key Takeaway:
The large intestine is more than a waste pipe — it's a **command center for blood sugar and brain health.** The gut microbiome influences insulin, cravings, memory, and mood. Your vivid dream and taste episodes before bowel movements are likely part of this **gut–brain signaling loop.**

PRACTICAL EATING TIPS FOR BLOOD SUGAR BALANCE

1. **Chew slowly.** Aim for 20–30 chews per bite, especially with carbs.
2. **Eat in order:** Veggies first → protein/fats → carbs last.
3. **Pause between bites.** Give saliva and enzymes time to work.
4. **Hydrate between meals, not during.** Too much liquid with meals can dilute stomach acids.
5. **Don't skip fiber.** It's the broom for your bowels *and* the buffer for your bloodstream.

Key Takeaway: Digestion starts before food ever hits your stomach. The way you chew, the order you eat, and the fiber you include all control how much sugar ends up flooding your bloodstream — and ultimately, how your brain and pancreas respond.

Water Intake & Blood Sugar Balance

WHY WATER MATTERS

- Glucose is carried in your blood — and blood is mostly water.
- When you're dehydrated, your blood sugar **concentrates**, meaning even normal glucose amounts read as higher.
- Water also helps your **kidneys flush out excess sugar** through urine, lowering blood glucose naturally.

HOW MUCH WATER? (GENERAL RULE)

- **Baseline:** 8–10 cups (2–2.5 L) per day for most adults.
- **More if:** hot weather, exercise, fever, or high blood sugar (since sugar draws water out of tissues).
- **Best practice:** Spread throughout the day, not all at once.

BEST TIMING FOR HYDRATION

1. **Morning (on waking):** 1–2 cups → rehydrates after overnight.
2. **Before meals:** 1 glass ~15–30 minutes before eating → supports digestion, prevents overeating.
3. **After carb-heavy meals:** A glass of water helps the kidneys flush extra glucose.
4. **Evening:** Light sipping only → too much before bed disrupts sleep with bathroom trips.

BY DIABETES TYPE
Type 1 Diabetes

- **Why water matters:** High blood sugars cause the kidneys to pull water into urine (polyuria = frequent urination). Dehydration can happen fast.
- **Goal:** Regular, steady hydration throughout the day.
- **Caution:** Excessive thirst and urination may signal poor glucose control (hyperglycemia) or dangerous complications (like diabetic ketoacidosis).
- **Tip:** If you're suddenly *very* thirsty all the time → check blood sugar immediately.

Type 2 Diabetes

- **Why water matters:** Proper hydration lowers fasting glucose and reduces insulin resistance.
- **Goal:** 8–12 cups/day, more if blood sugar is running high.
- **Tip:** Drinking water before meals can cut post-meal glucose spikes by 20–30%.
- **Caution:** Constant, excessive thirst (polydipsia) may be a warning sign of chronically high blood sugar.

Type 3 Diabetes (Sugar–Brain Connection)

- **Why water matters:** The brain is 75% water; dehydration worsens brain fog, memory lapses, and mood swings.
- **Goal:** Consistent hydration (small sips often), not big gulps.
- **Tip:** Herbal teas (cinnamon, ginger, green tea) hydrate while supporting blood sugar and the brain.
- **Caution:** Overhydrating can dilute electrolytes → leading to dizziness, confusion, or worsening brain symptoms.

What About Drinking Too Much Water?

Drinking **excessive amounts** (like >4–5 L/day without medical need) can backfire:

- **Dilutes sodium & electrolytes** (hyponatremia) →
  headaches, nausea, confusion, even seizures.
- **Kidney strain:** Kidneys can only filter so much water
  per hour (~1 L). Beyond that, excess flushes electrolytes
  too quickly.
- **Clue:** If your urine is completely clear *all day long*, you
  may be overhydrating. Healthy hydration = light yellow.

Practical Hydration Hacks

- Carry a refillable bottle (but pace yourself, not
  chugging).
- Add lemon, cucumber, or mint for flavor.
- Use **herbal teas** as part of hydration.
- Pair water with electrolytes (like a pinch of sea salt or
  mineral drops) if drinking >3 L/day.
- Track thirst + urination: sudden changes often = blood
  sugar shifts.

Key Takeaway:

- **Type 1:** Hydration is a safety net — dehydration
  worsens risks. Watch for excessive thirst.
- **Type 2:** Water lowers insulin resistance and curbs post-
  meal spikes.
- **Type 3:** Hydration supports the brain, but overhydration
  can worsen fog by diluting electrolytes.

Types of Sugar & What They Do to the Body

1. GLUCOSE (THE BODY'S PRIMARY SUGAR)

- Found naturally in fruit, honey, and starchy foods.
- Directly enters the bloodstream → raises blood sugar **quickly.**
- Needed by every cell for energy, especially the brain.
- Excess → insulin surge, fat storage, cravings.

Impact: All diabetics must monitor glucose; stable intake is key.

- **Type 1:**
  - o Directly raises blood sugar — must be carefully matched with insulin.
  - o Needed quickly if blood sugar goes too low (glucose tabs or juice = lifesaving).
- **Type 2:**
  - o Spikes blood sugar quickly, requiring more insulin.
  - o Worsens insulin resistance over time.
- **Type 3 (Brain link):**
  - o The brain depends on glucose, but unstable delivery (spikes + crashes) = brain fog, memory lapses, panic feelings.

2. FRUCTOSE (FRUIT SUGAR)

- Found in fruit, honey, agave, and high-fructose corn syrup (HFCS).
- Processed by the **liver, not directly by insulin.**
- Small amounts (from whole fruit) = fine (comes with fiber + antioxidants).

- Large amounts (soda, sweeteners, HFCS) = liver overload → fatty liver, insulin resistance.

Impact:

- **Type 1:** Still affects blood sugar, though slower.
- **Type 2 & 3:** Dangerous in excess → worsens insulin resistance & fatty liver.

- **Type 1:**

  - Still raises blood sugar (though slower than glucose).
  - Must still be counted for insulin dosing.

- **Type 2:**

  - Processed mostly in the liver → contributes to **fatty liver disease** and worsens insulin resistance.
  - High-fructose corn syrup (HFCS) in soda = especially dangerous.

- **Type 3:**

  - Too much fructose increases **brain inflammation** and may worsen dementia risk.
  - Whole fruit with fiber = okay (berries best).

3. SUCROSE (TABLE SUGAR)

- 50% glucose + 50% fructose.
- Found in cane sugar, brown sugar, and processed foods.
- Raises blood sugar quickly **and** strains the liver.

Impact: Main culprit in sugar spikes, crashes, and long-term insulin resistance.

- **Type 1:** Rapid spike → insulin required. Best avoided outside of emergencies.
- **Type 2:** Double trouble: raises glucose **and** strains the liver.
- **Type 3:** Sharp spikes + inflammatory fructose load = brain fog, cravings, memory dips.

4. LACTOSE (MILK SUGAR)

- Found in milk and dairy.
- Requires the enzyme **lactase** to be digested (many adults lack enough, leading to bloating/gas).
- Moderately raises blood sugar.
- Dairy products like cheese and Greek yogurt have **very little lactose** → better tolerated.

Impact: Not as dangerous as refined sugars, but still a carb source.

• **Type 1:** Raises blood sugar moderately; must be accounted for in carb counts.

• **Type 2:** Generally moderate effect, but lactose intolerance is more common and can add GI stress.

• **Type 3:** Dairy with protein (like Greek yogurt, cottage cheese) can stabilize blood sugar, but milk or sweetened dairy (ice cream, flavored yogurt) can worsen crashes.

5. MALTOSE & STARCHES

- Found in malted foods (beer, cereals, pretzels).
- Starches (white bread, rice, pasta, potatoes) break down into maltose → glucose.
- High-glycemic, meaning very quick spikes.

Impact: Behaves just like sugar in the bloodstream — especially problematic for **Type 2 & 3.**

- **Type 1:** Spike blood sugar fast — must match insulin carefully.
- **Type 2:** Behave like sugar; constant starch-heavy meals drive insulin resistance.
- **Type 3:** Major culprit for brain fog episodes, memory blanks, and vivid dream "crashes."

TYPES OF SUGAR SUBSTITUTES
Natural Low/No-Calorie Sweeteners

Stevia

- Plant-based, zero-calorie, doesn't raise blood sugar.
- Can have a bitter aftertaste for some.
- Safe for all diabetes types.

Monk Fruit

- Plant-based, zero-calorie, doesn't raise blood sugar.
- Often blended with other sweeteners (check label).

Allulose

- Rare sugar, almost zero calories.
- Doesn't spike blood sugar, may even improve insulin sensitivity.

Erythritol (sugar alcohol)

- Almost calorie-free, very low impact on blood sugar.
- Some people experience bloating or gas if consumed in large amounts.

CAUTION SWEETENERS

Xylitol (sugar alcohol)

- Low glycemic, doesn't spike blood sugar much.
- BUT can cause bloating or diarrhea in sensitive people.
- **Toxic to dogs** — must be kept away from pets.

Agave syrup

- Marketed as healthy, but up to **90% fructose.**
- Overloads the liver → increases insulin resistance.
- Worse than table sugar for many diabetics.

ARTIFICIAL SWEETENERS (LAB-MADE)

Aspartame (Equal)

- Found in diet sodas, sugar-free gum.
- Doesn't raise blood sugar, but may alter brain chemistry and worsen cravings for sweets.

Sucralose (Splenda)

- Can spike insulin even without calories.
- Alters gut microbiome in some people.

Saccharin

- One of the oldest artificial sweeteners.
- Not absorbed in the gut, but may alter microbiome.

Impact: Artificial sweeteners don't spike blood sugar directly, but they can **trick the brain** into craving more carbs and disrupt gut health.

SUGAR SUBSTITUTES: BY TYPE

Stevia, Monk Fruit, Allulose

- **Type 1:** Don't raise blood sugar — safe.
- **Type 2:** Help reduce sugar intake, lower cravings.
- **Type 3:** Brain-friendly (no spikes, no crashes).

Sugar Alcohols (erythritol, xylitol, sorbitol)

- **Type 1:** Minimal impact, but large amounts can cause GI distress.
- **Type 2:** Low glycemic; helpful but should be in moderation.
- **Type 3:** Can worsen gut imbalance if overused (gut-brain link).

Artificial Sweeteners (aspartame, sucralose, saccharin)

- **Type 1:** Don't raise blood sugar, but may trick the appetite and affect gut health.
- **Type 2:** Some studies suggest they worsen insulin resistance over time.
- **Type 3:** May trigger cravings and alter brain chemistry — best limited.

Agave Syrup, HFCS, Cane Sugar

- **Type 1:** Strong blood sugar spikes, insulin required.
- **Type 2:** Worst offenders for insulin resistance and fatty liver.
- **Type 3:** Fuel brain inflammation and memory decline — best avoided.

BEST CHOICE FOR BLOOD SUGAR BALANCE

- **Whole fruit (in moderation, with fiber)** → best natural sweetness.
- **Stevia, monk fruit, erythritol, allulose** → safest substitutes for diabetics.
- **Avoid:** Agave, HFCS, large amounts of honey/maple syrup, and artificial sweeteners if possible.

Key Takeaway:
Not all sugars are equal. **Glucose fuels, fructose strains, sucrose spikes, starches mimic sugar.** For sweeteners, choose natural low-glycemic options like **stevia, monk fruit, or allulose.**

Herbs for Blood Sugar & Brain Health (by Type)

TYPE 1 DIABETES

(*Insulin-dependent: herbs may support overall health, but never replace insulin*)
Focus: inflammation reduction, antioxidant support, stable digestion.

- **Cinnamon** – May lower post-meal glucose, but the effect is modest; can be a safe add-on with insulin.
- **Fenugreek seeds** – Slow carb absorption and may improve post-meal spikes.
- **Aloe vera juice (unsweetened)** – Anti-inflammatory; may improve fasting glucose.
- **Turmeric/Curcumin** – Reduces inflammation that worsens diabetic complications.
- **Milk thistle** – Liver support; may aid blood sugar regulation.

Caution: Herbs can lower blood sugar → risk of hypoglycemia if combined with insulin. Always monitor closely.

TYPE 2 DIABETES

(*Insulin resistance: herbs can improve sensitivity, reduce spikes, and support weight loss*)
Focus: insulin sensitivity, lowering fasting glucose, reducing inflammation.

- **Cinnamon** – Improves insulin sensitivity, reduces fasting glucose.
- **Berberine** – Powerful; shown to be as effective as metformin in some studies (supports gut health + lowers glucose).

- **Gymnema sylvestre** ("sugar destroyer") – Reduces sugar absorption in the gut and cravings for sweets.
- **Fenugreek** – Supports better blood sugar control; also improves cholesterol.
- **Bitter melon** – Mimics insulin activity, lowers glucose.
- **Green tea (catechins)** – Improves insulin sensitivity and supports fat burning.
- **Ginger** – Lowers inflammation and may help reduce A1c.

Caution: Combining strong herbs (berberine, bitter melon, gymnema) with meds can cause hypoglycemia — must be monitored.

TYPE 3 DIABETES (SUGAR–BRAIN CONNECTION, ALZHEIMER'S LINK)

(Focus: brain protection, reducing sugar floods, improving memory and neurotransmitter balance)

- **Turmeric/Curcumin** – Protects neurons, reduces amyloid plaque formation, and lowers inflammation.
- **Sage** – Improves memory, cognitive performance, and focus.
- **Rosemary** – Enhances circulation to the brain, improves memory.
- **Gotu Kola** – Traditional brain tonic; supports microcirculation in the brain.
- **Ginkgo biloba** – Increases blood flow to the brain; supports memory and attention.
- **Green tea** – Antioxidants protect brain cells; supports steady energy.
- **Cinnamon** – Stabilizes blood sugar, reduces brain glucose swings.
- **Ashwagandha** – Lowers cortisol (stress hormone that spikes blood sugar).

Caution: Many brain herbs thin the blood slightly (like ginkgo, rosemary), so they should be avoided with certain meds or if surgery is upcoming.

PRACTICAL HERB USE TIPS

- **Start low and slow.** Herbs are medicine, not just "spices."
- **Choose teas or capsules.** Cinnamon tea, turmeric lattes, fenugreek tea, and green tea are easy daily options.
- **Rotate herbs.** Don't rely on just one — variety improves benefits and prevents overuse.
- **Monitor closely.** Especially with Type 1 or Type 2 on meds — herbs may lower glucose further.

KEY TAKEAWAY:

- **Type 1:** Herbs = supportive (anti-inflammatory, gentle stabilizers), but insulin is still essential.
- **Type 2:** Herbs can be powerful tools to improve insulin sensitivity and lower spikes.
- **Type 3:** Brain-protective herbs (turmeric, sage, rosemary, ginkgo) + stabilizers (cinnamon, green tea) are most helpful.

Natural Supports for Blood Sugar

1. CEYLON CINNAMON ("TRUE CINNAMON")

- **What it is:** A spice from the inner bark of the Ceylon tree (different from the common Cassia cinnamon).
- **How it works:**
  - Improves **insulin sensitivity** → cells respond better to insulin.
  - May slow stomach emptying → steadier glucose release.
  - Adds sweetness without sugar → helpful for cravings.
- **Best for:**
  - **Type 2 & Type 3:** Reduces fasting glucose, lowers A1c slightly.
  - **Type 1:** Mild benefit but not a substitute for insulin.
- **Caution:** Cassia cinnamon (the cheaper grocery store kind) contains **coumarin**, which in high doses can stress the liver. Ceylon is safer for daily use.

2. BERBERINE

- **What it is:** A compound found in plants like barberry, goldenseal, and Oregon grape.
- **How it works:**
  - Activates **AMPK** ("the metabolic master switch") → improves insulin sensitivity and fat metabolism.
  - Reduces glucose production in the liver.
  - Shown in studies to lower A1c by **up to 1%** (similar to metformin).
- **Best for:**
  - **Type 2:** Strongest evidence — helps with insulin resistance and weight control.

- o **Type 3:** May protect brain cells by reducing inflammation and oxidative stress.
- **Caution:**
  - o Can interact with medications (especially metformin, statins, and blood pressure meds).
  - o May cause digestive upset if the dose is too high.

3. CHROMIUM

- **What it is:** A trace mineral needed in tiny amounts.
- **How it works:**
  - o Helps **insulin bind more effectively** to cells.
  - o Reduces cravings for carbs and sugar.
  - o Supports energy metabolism.
- **Best for:**
  - o **Type 2:** May lower fasting glucose and improve cholesterol.
  - o **Type 3:** Steadier insulin activity = steadier brain fuel.
- **Caution:**
  - o Deficiency is rare, but supplementation can help if the diet is poor.
  - o Too much chromium can cause kidney or liver strain — stay within safe doses (200–1000 mcg/day).

4. BITTER MELON

- **What it is:** A tropical gourd-like fruit used in Asian and African traditional medicine.
- **How it works:**
  - o Contains **charantin** and **polypeptide-p**, which mimic insulin.
  - o Helps cells absorb glucose more effectively.
  - o Lowers fasting glucose and post-meal spikes.
- **Best for:**
  - o **Type 2:** Especially useful for insulin resistance.

- o **Type 3:** May reduce brain fog by stabilizing blood sugar swings.
- **Caution:**
  - o Can cause hypoglycemia if combined with medications.
  - o Avoid during pregnancy (stimulates the uterus).
  - o Very bitter taste — best as tea, capsule, or cooked dish.

5. TURMERIC (CURCUMIN)

- **What it is:** A bright yellow spice from the turmeric root, widely used in Indian cooking and medicine.
- **How it works:**
  - o Strong **anti-inflammatory** and **antioxidant.**
  - o Protects pancreatic cells from damage.
  - o May reduce insulin resistance.
  - o Protects brain cells (reduces amyloid plaque buildup → Alzheimer's prevention).
- **Best for:**
  - o **Type 2:** Supports insulin sensitivity.
  - o **Type 3:** Protects neurons, improves memory, and mood.
- **Caution:**
  - o Works best with black pepper (piperine) for absorption.
  - o Can interact with blood thinners and gallbladder issues.

Key Takeaway Summary

- **Ceylon Cinnamon:** Gentle stabilizer, safe daily.
- **Berberine:** Powerful, comparable to metformin — best for Type 2.
- **Chromium:** Mineral helper, good for carb cravings and insulin efficiency.

- **Bitter Melon:** Insulin mimic, strong effect but bitter taste.
- **Turmeric:** Anti-inflammatory, protects the pancreas and brain (especially for Type 3).

Natural Supports for the Brain

ROSEMARY (ROSMARINUS OFFICINALIS)
Traditional Uses

- Called the "herb of remembrance" since ancient Greece and Rome.
- Students in Greece wore rosemary sprigs while studying to improve memory.
- Used in medieval times to protect against "mental fog" and melancholy.

How It Works (Modern Science)

- **Carnosic acid & rosmarinic acid** (antioxidants) → protect neurons from free-radical damage.
- Improves **cerebral circulation** → more blood and oxygen to the brain.
- May inhibit amyloid plaque formation (linked to Alzheimer's).
- Enhances acetylcholine (a neurotransmitter for learning and memory).

For Diabetes & Brain Health

- Helps counter the "starved neuron" problem of brain insulin resistance.
- Supports sharper memory, alertness, and focus (great for brain fog days).
- Anti-inflammatory effects may reduce the risk of cognitive decline.

How to Use

- **Tea:** Steep 1 tsp dried rosemary or a fresh sprig in hot water for 10 min.
- **Culinary:** Use fresh rosemary in roasted veggies, meats, and soups.
- **Aromatherapy:** Rosemary essential oil inhalation improves short-term memory and alertness.

Cautions

- Avoid very high doses (may irritate the stomach or increase blood pressure).
- Essential oils should never be ingested, only inhaled or diluted for topical use.

SAGE (SALVIA OFFICINALIS)
Traditional Uses

- The name comes from *salvare* (Latin = "to save").
- Historically used for wisdom, longevity, and calming the mind.
- In European herbal medicine, sage was brewed to sharpen memory and soothe nerves.

How It Works (Modern Science)

- Contains compounds that **inhibit acetylcholinesterase** — the same mechanism as some Alzheimer's drugs (it keeps more acetylcholine available in the brain).
- Antioxidants reduce oxidative stress on neurons.
- May improve mood and reduce anxiety (balancing neurotransmitters).

For Diabetes & Brain Health

- Improves memory, learning, and attention in both healthy adults and Alzheimer's patients (studies show measurable cognitive improvements after sage extract).
- Helps regulate blood sugar by improving insulin sensitivity.
- Reduces inflammation that contributes to both diabetes and dementia.

How to Use

- **Tea:** Steep 1 tsp dried sage leaves (or a few fresh) in hot water for 5–10 min.
- **Culinary:** Add to soups, stews, meats, or roasted vegetables.
- **Supplements:** Sage extract capsules (often standardized for clinical effects).

- **Aromatherapy:** Sage essential oil may improve mood, but use diluted.

Cautions

- In very high doses, sage contains thujone (can be toxic) — normal tea/culinary use is safe.
- Avoid concentrated essential oil internally.

Why These Herbs Matter for Type 3 Diabetes

- **Rosemary** = improves brain circulation + antioxidant defense.
- **Sage** = boosts memory chemicals (acetylcholine) + balances blood sugar.
- Together, they **protect the diabetic brain** from both short-term fog and long-term decline.

HERBAL & NUTRIENT CHEAT SHEET FOR BLOOD SUGAR & BRAIN HEALTH

Herb/ Nutrient	What It Does	Best For	How to Take	Cautions
Ceylon Cinnamon	Improves insulin sensitivity, slows stomach emptying, reduces cravings	Type 2 & 3 (mild help in Type 1)	½–1 tsp daily in tea, smoothies, or food	Use Ceylon, not Cassia (Cassia has coumarin → liver risk in high doses)
Berberine	Activates AMPK (metabolic switch), lowers fasting glucose, reduces liver sugar production	Type 2 (insulin resistance), Type 3 (neuroprotection)	500 mg, 2–3x/day with meals	May cause digestive upset; interacts with metformin, statins, BP meds
Chromium	Helps insulin bind to cells, reduces carb/sugar cravings	Type 2 & 3 (steadier brain fuel)	200–1000 mcg/day (as chromium picolinate)	Too much can strain kidneys/liver; avoid megadoses
Bitter Melon	Mimics insulin, improves	Type 2 & 3 (brain fog	Tea: ½ fruit sliced & steeped;	Can cause hypoglycemia with

Herb/ Nutrient	What It Does	Best For	How to Take	Cautions
	glucose uptake, lowers post-meal spikes	from sugar swings)	Capsules: 500–1000 mg/day	meds; avoid in pregnancy
Turmeric *Curcumin*	Anti-inflammatory, protects pancreatic cells, improves memory, reduces amyloid plaque	Type 2 (insulin sensitivity), Type 3 (brain health)	500–1000 mg curcumin/ day + black pepper, or as golden milk/tea	Avoid if on blood thinners; can worsen gallbladder issues
Rosemary	Improves brain circulation, protects neurons with antioxidants, may slow plaque buildup	Type 3 (memory, brain fog, dementia prevention)	Tea (1 tsp dried or fresh sprig steeped), in cooking, or aromatherapy	Avoid very high doses; essential oil not for internal use
Sage	Boosts memory & focus (preserves	Type 2 & 3 (cognitive clarity, mood balance)	Tea (1 tsp dried leaves), culinary use, or	High doses contain thujone (toxic); avoid

Herb/ Nutrient	What It Does	Best For	How to Take	Cautions
	acetylcho line), reduces anxiety, supports blood sugar control		standardiz ed extract	internal use of essential oil

Movement as Medicine

Most people think of exercise as something you do at the gym: sweating, lifting, running, or following a structured routine. But when it comes to blood sugar balance, even **simple, gentle movement** can be as effective as some medications.

WHY MOVEMENT MATTERS FOR BLOOD SUGAR

When you move, your muscles act like sponges, soaking up glucose from the bloodstream. This process happens **without needing as much insulin**, which gives your pancreas a much-needed break. Over time, this reduces insulin resistance and helps your body manage sugar more efficiently.

Think of it this way:

- **Sitting after a meal** = sugar stays in the bloodstream longer.
- **Moving after a meal** = muscles pull sugar out of the bloodstream and use it for fuel.

WALKING AFTER MEALS – THE SECRET WEAPON

Research has shown that something as simple as a **10–15 minute walk after eating** can lower post-meal blood sugar spikes as effectively as certain medications prescribed for Type 2 diabetes.

Why? Because:

- Walking directly uses the sugar from the meal you just ate.
- It prevents the "sugar flood" from overwhelming your system.

- It supports digestion and reduces that heavy, sluggish feeling after eating.

OTHER TYPES OF MOVEMENT THAT HELP

- **Strength Training:** Builds muscle, which increases the body's long-term ability to burn glucose.
- **Yoga & Stretching:** Reduces stress hormones (which otherwise raise blood sugar) and improves circulation.
- **Low-Impact Cardio:** Cycling, swimming, or dancing keeps blood sugar stable without over-stressing the body.
- **Everyday Movement:** Gardening, cleaning, or even standing up and pacing during a phone call all count.

THE TAKEAWAY

Movement isn't about burning calories—it's about **using glucose efficiently** and **taking the load off your pancreas.** You don't need to overhaul your life or join a gym to see benefits. Just walking after meals, moving regularly throughout the day, and adding small bursts of activity can create profound changes in blood sugar stability.

GENTLE VS. VIGOROUS EXERCISE

When it comes to blood sugar, **gentle movement can sometimes be more effective than vigorous workouts.**

- **Gentle Movement (walking, yoga, light cycling):**
    - Uses glucose steadily during and after activity.
    - Is sustainable and doesn't spike stress hormones.
    - Perfect for post-meal walks, daily routines, and calming the nervous system.
- **Vigorous Exercise (running, HIIT, heavy cardio):**

o Burns more energy, but also raises cortisol (stress hormone), which can temporarily raise blood sugar.
o Still valuable, especially for heart health and fitness, but not always the best choice if you're highly insulin resistant or prone to crashes.
o Works best when layered onto a foundation of gentle, daily activity.

The key isn't pushing harder—it's **moving consistently**. For many people with diabetes or prediabetes, 10–15 minutes of walking after meals has more blood sugar impact than 60 minutes of intense gym workouts.

HOW EXERCISE REDUCES BRAIN RISK TOO

Movement isn't just about muscles and blood sugar—it's also powerful **protection for the brain.**

- **Increases Insulin Sensitivity in the Brain:** Regular exercise improves how brain cells use glucose, reducing the risk of brain fog, memory lapses, and cognitive decline linked to Type 3 diabetes.
- **Boosts Blood Flow:** Movement improves circulation, carrying oxygen and nutrients directly to brain tissue.
- **Stimulates Neuroplasticity:** Exercise triggers the release of BDNF (Brain-Derived Neurotrophic Factor), often called "fertilizer for the brain," which helps neurons grow and connect.
- **Lowers Inflammation:** Chronic inflammation is tied to both insulin resistance and brain aging. Movement helps keep inflammation in check.

THE TAKEAWAY

Exercise is a two-for-one gift: it balances blood sugar **and** lowers your risk of cognitive decline. You don't need perfection—you just need consistency. A short walk after meals, gentle stretching in the evening, or even gardening can be as healing for your brain as they are for your body.

WHEN EXERCISE DOESN'T "WORK" THE WAY YOU EXPECT

I once committed to exercising three to five times a week for an entire year. I worked hard, I ate better, I expected the pounds to fall away. Instead? I lost just three pounds. Frustrating doesn't even begin to cover it.

So why does this happen?

1. Exercise Improves Blood Sugar First, Not Always Weight

2. Insulin Resistance Can Stall Weight Loss

3. Stress & Hormones Can Override Exercise

4. The Brain Connection (Type 3)

IN MORE DEPTH: 1. EXERCISE IMPROVES BLOOD SUGAR FIRST, NOT ALWAYS WEIGHT

When you move, your muscles become active sugar sponges. They pull glucose out of your bloodstream and use it for energy — a process that can happen **even without insulin.** This is huge, because it means exercise gives your pancreas a break and helps reset your cells' responsiveness to insulin.

But here's the important truth:

- These shifts in blood sugar and insulin sensitivity often happen **long before the scale changes.**
- Your blood sugar may be stabilizing, your brain may be clearer, and your energy may be steadier — even if your weight hasn't budged.

Think of it like **repair work inside your house**: the plumbing and wiring may be getting fixed, but you won't notice the changes until later, when the lights turn on and the water runs smoothly. Exercise is repairing your inner wiring before you see changes on the outside.

WHY THE SCALE MAY NOT MOVE QUICKLY

1. **Blood Sugar Comes First** – Your body prioritizes healing glucose control over dropping pounds.
2. **Muscle vs. Fat** – Exercise builds lean muscle, which weighs more than fat but burns more sugar long term.
3. **Cortisol & Stress** – If your system is inflamed or stressed (common in insulin resistance), cortisol can block weight loss even if exercise is helping in other ways.
4. **Type of Diabetes Matters** – The way your body responds to movement depends on whether it's Type 1, Type 2, or Type 3.

EXERCISE & THE TYPES OF DIABETES
Type 1 Diabetes

- In Type 1, the pancreas produces little to no insulin. Exercise still lowers blood sugar, but people with Type 1 need to be especially careful: too much activity without adjusting insulin or eating can cause dangerous hypoglycemia.

For them, exercise is about **balance and safety** — pairing movement with careful glucose monitoring.

Type 2 Diabetes

- In Type 2, the body makes insulin, but the cells resist it. Exercise is one of the most powerful tools here:
  - Muscles absorb glucose directly, bypassing some of that insulin resistance.

    o   Regular movement retrains cells to be more insulin-sensitive.
- For many with Type 2, exercise can be as effective as medication in lowering A1C and improving long-term glucose control.

Type 3 Diabetes (The Sugar–Brain Connection)

- In Type 3, insulin resistance extends to the brain. The brain cells don't use glucose efficiently, leading to brain fog, memory issues, and a higher risk of Alzheimer's.
- Exercise is crucial because it:
  - Improves insulin sensitivity in the brain, not just the body.
  - Boosts blood flow and oxygen to brain tissue.
  - Stimulates **BDNF** (Brain-Derived Neurotrophic Factor), which helps brain cells grow, repair, and connect — like fertilizer for your neurons.
- For Type 3, movement isn't just about lowering blood sugar — it's literally **protecting your memory, mood, and long-term brain health.**

THE REAL PAYOFF OF MOVEMENT

- **Immediate:** steadier post-meal blood sugar, fewer spikes and crashes.
- **Short Term (weeks to months):** improved insulin sensitivity, reduced brain fog, more consistent energy.
- **Long Term (years):** lower risk of complications like heart disease, neuropathy, and cognitive decline.

Even if the scale is slow to respond, your body is **already healing and protecting itself** every time you move.

2. INSULIN RESISTANCE CAN STALL WEIGHT LOSS

In Type 2 and especially Type 3 diabetes, your body is dealing with **insulin resistance** — meaning your cells aren't listening properly to insulin's signal. Normally, insulin acts like a key, unlocking your cells so glucose (sugar) can get inside and be used as fuel. But when resistance sets in, the "lock" is jammed.

That means:

- Glucose lingers in the bloodstream instead of being burned for energy.
- The pancreas pumps out even more insulin, trying to force the door open.
- Excess insulin in the blood sends a message to your body: **"Store this energy as fat."**

This is why, even if you're eating better and exercising regularly, the scale may not budge — your body is literally wired to **hold onto fat** when insulin resistance is in play.

THE SUGAR–BRAIN LINK (TYPE 3 TWIST)

With Type 3, insulin resistance doesn't just affect your muscles and fat cells — it affects your **brain cells** too. When neurons can't use glucose efficiently, your brain sends confusing signals about hunger, cravings, and fullness:

- You may feel hungrier than you "should."
- Carbs and sweets might call to you more strongly.
- Your brain may tell your body to store fat even when you're trying to burn it.

It's not a lack of willpower — it's your brain chemistry reacting to insulin resistance.

WHY EXERCISE ALONE ISN'T ENOUGH

Exercise helps, but if insulin resistance is strong, your cells may still ignore insulin's signal. That's why weight loss can be painfully slow, even when you're doing "everything right." The truth is:

- **Food quality & balance** (protein, healthy fats, fiber-rich carbs) matter just as much as exercise.
- **Stress reduction** lowers cortisol, which makes insulin resistance worse.
- **Sleep quality** affects how sensitive your cells are to insulin.

ENCOURAGING PERSPECTIVE

If you've ever felt like your body was working against you — you're right, in a way. Insulin resistance sets up a biochemical traffic jam. But here's the hope: every time you eat a balanced meal, take a walk, or reduce stress, you're slowly clearing that traffic. Over time, the signals get clearer, and your body begins to shift from storing to burning.

THE TRUTH ABOUT EXERCISE AND WEIGHT

Exercise is medicine—but it's not a magic weight-loss pill. Its greatest gift is helping your muscles and brain use sugar more efficiently, reducing stress on your pancreas, and protecting your brain from the long-term effects of high blood sugar.

The real shift comes when **exercise + balanced meals + stress management + sleep** all line up. That's when weight and energy often begin to improve more noticeably.

PERSONAL NOTE

Looking back, I realize my exercise wasn't wasted at all. Even if the scale barely moved, my body was still repairing itself beneath the surface. My blood sugar was steadier, my energy was better, and I was giving my pancreas and brain some relief. The weight-loss story is just one piece of the puzzle—and often the slowest one to show up.

3. STRESS & HORMONES CAN OVERRIDE EXERCISE

You can be eating better, walking daily, even hitting the gym — and still not see results if your stress hormones are in overdrive. The biggest culprit? **Cortisol.**

Cortisol is your body's primary stress hormone. It's designed to give you quick energy in emergencies (the classic "fight or flight" response). But when blood sugar is already spiking and crashing, cortisol stays elevated — and that creates a vicious cycle.

HOW CORTISOL AFFECTS BLOOD SUGAR AND WEIGHT

- **Raises Blood Sugar:** Cortisol signals your liver to release stored glucose into the bloodstream, giving your body an emergency energy boost. If you're not actually fighting or fleeing, that sugar just lingers — and often ends up stored as fat.
- **Increases Insulin Resistance:** High cortisol makes your cells even less responsive to insulin, forcing your pancreas to pump out more.
- **Promotes Belly Fat Storage:** Cortisol specifically encourages fat storage around the midsection — the

most dangerous kind linked to Type 2 and Type 3 diabetes.

- **Messes with Hunger Hormones:** Cortisol raises ghrelin (the hunger hormone), lowers leptin (the fullness hormone), and makes cravings for sugar and carbs much stronger.

WHY EXERCISE ALONE CAN'T UNDO STRESS HORMONES

If you're stuck in a stress cycle, exercise may not lower blood sugar or weight as effectively because cortisol is still telling your body to hold on to fat. In fact, overly **intense exercise** (like high-intensity workouts when your body is already stressed) can make things worse by spiking cortisol even higher.

This is why someone can say, *"I exercise and eat well, but I'm still gaining weight"* — the stress–cortisol–insulin triangle is overpowering their efforts.

PRACTICAL WAYS TO BREAK THE STRESS CYCLE

- **Gentle movement**: Walking, yoga, stretching, tai chi — lowers cortisol without spiking it.
- **Deep breathing & meditation**: Even 5 minutes can calm your nervous system and reduce stress hormone output.
- **Sleep hygiene**: Poor sleep raises cortisol the next day; consistent bedtime routines help regulate hormones.
- **Laughter & joy**: Cortisol's antidote is oxytocin and endorphins. Even simple pleasures (a funny show, time with loved ones, a hobby) reduce stress hormones.
- **Balanced meals**: Preventing blood sugar crashes lowers the "emergency alarm" that triggers cortisol in the first place.

PERSONAL REFLECTION

Looking back, I realize some of my most frustrating blood sugar days weren't about what I ate or how much I moved. They were about stress. Those nights of panic-like episodes, the brain fog, even the sudden hunger — my body wasn't just out of balance, it was in **alarm mode.** Learning to calm my nervous system was just as important as walking after dinner.

Stress, Sleep & Spirit

Balancing blood sugar isn't just about food and movement. Stress, sleep, and even your spiritual life play a massive role. You can be eating well and walking daily, but if your stress hormones are surging or your sleep is disrupted, your blood sugar will still rise and fall unpredictably.

STRESS HORMONES AND BLOOD SUGAR

Your body was designed with an ancient survival system: when danger strikes, stress hormones flood your bloodstream to prepare you for action.

- **Cortisol** is your long-term stress hormone. It raises blood sugar slowly and steadily, keeping energy available if the "threat" drags on.
- **Adrenaline (epinephrine)** is your short-term stress hormone. It spikes blood sugar fast, giving you an immediate burst of energy.

In a true emergency — like running from danger — this system works perfectly. Your muscles use the glucose surge, your body burns fuel, and the hormones calm down once the danger passes.

MODERN STRESS VS. ANCIENT BIOLOGY

The problem? Modern stress doesn't involve running or fighting. Instead of predators, our triggers are:

- A pile of bills you're worried about.
- A tense conversation at work.
- Waking in the night with anxious thoughts.
- Constant "noise" from phones, emails, and news.

Your brain doesn't know the difference. It still shouts **"Danger!"** and tells your liver: **"Dump sugar into the blood now!"**

But because you're sitting at your desk, lying in bed, or driving in your car, there's no physical outlet. The sugar isn't burned — it lingers in your bloodstream.

THE VICIOUS CYCLE

1. **Stress → Cortisol & Adrenaline Rise**
   Your liver releases glucose into the blood.
2. **Blood Sugar Spikes**
   If you're already insulin resistant, the sugar has nowhere to go.
3. **Pancreas Works Overtime**
   It releases more insulin to try to clear the sugar.
4. **Insulin Resistance Worsens**
   The more this cycle repeats, the harder it is for your cells to respond.
5. **The Brain Suffers**
   Constant sugar surges inflame the brain and disrupt hunger, mood, and memory.

This is how chronic stress directly fuels Type 2 diabetes, and why it's now being linked to **Type 3 (Alzheimer's and brain decline).**

EVERYDAY SIGNS STRESS IS SPIKING YOUR SUGAR

- You get shaky, sweaty, or ravenously hungry in the middle of a stressful day.
- You crash at 3 p.m. even though you ate lunch.
- You wake at 2–3 a.m. with your heart racing or mind racing.
- You crave sugar or carbs after an argument, deadline, or emotional day.

These aren't "bad habits" — they're **stress-driven blood sugar spikes.**

LONG-TERM WEAR AND TEAR

When this stress cycle repeats daily, it takes a toll:

- **Pancreas Burnout:** The pancreas can't keep up with constant insulin demands.
- **Fatigue:** Your body feels drained from adrenaline "false alarms."
- **Belly Fat Accumulation:** Cortisol promotes fat storage in the abdomen, the most harmful type.
- **Brain Changes:** Chronic stress shrinks the hippocampus (memory center) and weakens glucose use in brain cells, a hallmark of Type 3 diabetes.

WHY NIGHTTIME EPISODES HAPPEN

I learned this the hard way. My "night episodes" — the vivid dreams, the hyperventilation, the body trembling — were my brain and body crying out. When blood sugar dipped suddenly in the night, my stress hormones surged to rescue me. They jolted me awake with adrenaline, rapid breathing, and trembling — an internal alarm system trying to save me from a glucose crash.

This is why so many people with blood sugar imbalances struggle with:

- Waking at 2–3 a.m. with racing thoughts.
- Night sweats or trembling.
- Vivid dreams or panic-like awakenings.
- Exhaustion the next morning, even if they "slept."

It's not just bad luck or poor sleep habits. It's the **stress–blood sugar loop** playing out overnight.

SIMPLE TOOLS FOR CALMING STRESS & BALANCING BLOOD SUGAR

The good news: your nervous system can be retrained. Small daily practices calm stress hormones, which helps stabilize blood sugar and improve sleep.

- **Breathing:** Try the "4-7-8 method" (inhale 4, hold 7, exhale 8). This signals your body to drop out of fight-or-flight mode.
- **Meditation:** Even 5 minutes of quiet mindfulness lowers cortisol and steadies your heart rate.
- **Journaling:** Writing worries down before bed gets them out of your mind and reduces racing thoughts.
- **Prayer:** Connecting spiritually reduces anxiety and replaces fear with trust and peace.
- **Visualization:** Imagine your body as calm, steady, and nourished. Visualization can even help reduce nighttime episodes by preparing the brain to stay in rest mode.

THE SPIRIT CONNECTION

Stress and blood sugar aren't just physical battles — they're spiritual ones, too. Fear, worry, and self-blame spike your nervous system. But when you replace them with faith, gratitude, and inner peace, your body responds. Studies even show that prayer and spiritual practices lower blood pressure, improve sleep, and reduce stress hormones.

THE TAKEAWAY

Stress, sleep, and spirit are not "extras" — they are core parts of blood sugar balance. Healing isn't just about what you eat, but also how you breathe, rest, and connect to something bigger than yourself. When your body knows it's safe, it no longer needs to spike blood sugar as an emergency fuel.

4. THE BRAIN CONNECTION (TYPE 3)

When blood sugar is out of balance, it doesn't just affect your body — it scrambles the communication system inside your brain. Your brain runs almost entirely on glucose, but in **Type 3 diabetes (the sugar–brain connection)**, the cells can't use that fuel efficiently. The result? Your brain misreads hunger, energy, and memory signals.

HOW THE BRAIN MISFIRES WITH BLOOD SUGAR SWINGS

- **Hunger Signals Go Haywire:** Instead of a steady appetite, you get sudden, urgent cravings — usually for sugar or carbs.
- **Fullness Signals Get Confused:** You may eat a full meal but still feel like you need "something else" afterward.
- **Energy Crashes Hit Hard:** Instead of gradual tiredness, your brain suddenly feels drained, foggy, or panicked.
- **Mood Shifts:** Irritability, anxiety, or even panic can flare when your brain senses a shortage of glucose.

This isn't a lack of discipline or "being emotional." It's your brain chemistry **reacting to poor glucose delivery.**

WHY THIS MATTERS IN TYPE 3 DIABETES

- **Cognitive Decline:** Over time, poor glucose uptake by brain cells is linked to memory loss and Alzheimer's.
- **Brain Fog & Word Mix-Ups:** Forgetting why you walked into a room, losing your train of thought, or

mixing up words are all signs of glucose stress in the brain.

- **Exhaustion Despite Sleep:** You may sleep plenty but still wake up tired — because your brain didn't get steady fuel overnight.

PERSONAL REFLECTION

I used to think I was scatterbrained. Times when I'd go into a room and forget why I went there, or when I'd start to speak and lose the thought mid-sentence. Even as a teenager, I had shakiness and sudden hunger that made me *have* to eat. Later, when students or friends thought I was "high" or "buzzed" when I hadn't had a drink — it was actually my brain reacting to blood sugar swings.

Knowing this gave me freedom: it wasn't a character flaw, it was **chemistry.**

THE HOPEFUL SIDE

The good news is that this brain–sugar miscommunication isn't permanent. With stable blood sugar habits:

- Hunger and fullness cues normalize.
- Brain fog clears and memory sharpens.
- Cravings weaken because your brain isn't in "panic mode."
- Long-term, you protect your brain from decline.

Part IV – Living With Diabetes in the Real World

Urine & Diabetes: What Your Pee Can Tell You

1. HOW URINE WORKS (THE BASICS)

- The kidneys act as your body's **filters**.
- They remove waste, balance fluids, and decide what to keep (like glucose, electrolytes) and what to get rid of.
- Normally, urine is about **95% water** and 5% waste (urea, salts, small amounts of creatinine).

2. COLOR GUIDE: WHAT'S NORMAL, WHAT'S NOT

- **Pale yellow (straw-colored):**
  Ideal. Shows you're hydrated and your kidneys are working normally.
- **Clear (like water):**
  You may be *overhydrated* (flushing electrolytes) or drinking excessively — this sometimes happens in diabetes when high sugar makes you constantly thirsty.
- **Dark yellow/amber:**
  Sign of dehydration. Your kidneys are concentrating urine.
- **Orange/brown:** Possible liver/bile issue, dehydration, or certain meds.

- **Pink/red:** May be blood in the urine (infection, kidney stone, or other causes — needs medical check).
- **Foamy/bubbly:** May mean excess protein in urine — an early sign of kidney stress (important for diabetics).

3. HOW OFTEN SHOULD YOU PEE?

- **Normal:** 6–8 times/day.
- **More than 10+ times/day:** Could be overhydration, caffeine, or a sign of uncontrolled blood sugar (glucose pulling water with it).
- **Waking up more than once at night (nocturia):** Common in diabetes if blood sugar is high or kidneys are stressed.

4. DIABETES-SPECIFIC CLUES IN URINE

- **Sweet or fruity-smelling urine:**
  - o Caused by excess glucose being dumped.
  - o Classic diabetes sign (especially Type 1 or uncontrolled Type 2).
- **Frequent urination (polyuria):**
  - o High blood sugar pulls water into urine → constant bathroom trips.
  - o Leads to dehydration and fatigue.
- **Excessive thirst (polydipsia):**
  - o Follows polyuria — your body is trying to replace lost fluid.
- **Protein in urine (proteinuria):**
  - o Sign of kidney strain or early kidney disease (diabetic nephropathy).
- **Cloudy or foamy urine:**
  - o Possible infection (more common in diabetics).
  - o Or protein leakage.

5. THE KIDNEYS, SUGAR & RISK

- High blood sugar makes the kidneys **work overtime** filtering glucose.
- Over the years, this damages kidney blood vessels → **diabetic nephropathy.**
- Early detection: urine tests for **microalbumin** (tiny amounts of protein in urine).

6. WHAT TO DO FOR HEALTHY URINE & KIDNEYS

- **Hydrate wisely:** Water + herbal teas, not soda/juice.
- **Balance blood sugar:** Reduces glucose spillover into urine.
- **Monitor color:** Aim for pale yellow.
- **Get regular urine tests:** Check for protein, ketones, or infection.
- **Limit alcohol + processed salt:** Both stress the kidneys.
- **Herbal helpers:** Dandelion root tea (gentle diuretic), nettle leaf tea (supports kidneys).

7. SPECIAL NOTES BY TYPE

- **Type 1:** Watch for **ketones in urine** (can signal diabetic ketoacidosis — DKA — which is an emergency).
- **Type 2:** Frequent urination may be one of the first unnoticed symptoms; kidney strain is a long-term risk.
- **Type 3 (Brain connection):** Dehydration and electrolyte imbalances from excess urination can worsen **brain fog, vivid dreams, and memory issues.**

Key Takeaway:
Your urine is a free, daily lab test. Its color, smell, and frequency give valuable clues about hydration, blood sugar control, and kidney health. For anyone with diabetes — especially with the added brain connection of Type 3 —

keeping an eye on urine is one of the simplest ways to track what's happening inside the body.

Complications & Protection Strategies

Diabetes is often described in terms of numbers — glucose, A1c, and insulin. But what most people fear are the complications: nerve pain, vision loss, kidney failure, and heart disease.

Here's the good news: complications are not guaranteed. They are the *result of years of imbalance.* By learning how to protect your nerves, eyes, kidneys, and heart, you can reduce risk dramatically — and in many cases, prevent these problems altogether.

1. NEUROPATHY (NERVE DAMAGE)

What happens: High blood sugar damages the tiny blood vessels that feed nerves, especially in the feet and hands. This leads to numbness, tingling, pain, or weakness.

Protection Strategies:

- **Alpha-lipoic acid (ALA):** A powerful antioxidant that improves nerve blood flow and reduces pain.
- **Vitamin B12 (methylcobalamin):** Essential for the myelin sheath (nerve insulation). Deficiency is common in people taking metformin.
- **Reflexology & massage:** Improve circulation, stimulate nerves, and reduce discomfort.
- **Daily foot care:** Check for cuts or sores, wear well-fitting shoes, and moisturize.

2. RETINOPATHY (EYE DAMAGE)

What happens: Fragile blood vessels in the retina swell or leak, leading to blurry vision and, in severe cases, blindness.

Protection Strategies:

- **Lutein & zeaxanthin:** Carotenoids that concentrate in the retina and act as antioxidants. Found in leafy greens, egg yolks, and supplements.
- **Bilberry extract:** Improves microcirculation in the eyes.
- **Omega-3s (fish oil):** Reduce inflammation that damages vessels.
- **Eye yoga & breaks from screens:** Improve circulation and reduce strain.
- **Annual eye exams:** Detect problems early, before vision is affected.

3. KIDNEY STRESS (NEPHROPATHY)

What happens: The kidneys filter glucose along with waste. High blood sugar overworks them, leading to protein leakage and eventually kidney failure.

Protection Strategies:

- **Hydration:** Drink enough water to help flush toxins (urine pale yellow).
- **Nettle tea:** Traditional support for kidneys and urinary tract.
- **Balanced protein intake:** Too little = weakness, too much = kidney strain. Aim for moderate amounts, paired with fiber.
- **Avoid excess salt & processed foods:** Reduces kidney workload.

- **Regular urine tests:** Early detection of protein (microalbumin) allows intervention before damage.

4. HEART HEALTH (CARDIOVASCULAR DISEASE)

What happens: High sugar damages arteries, raising the risk of high blood pressure, heart attack, and stroke.

Protection Strategies:

- **Omega-3 fatty acids (fish, chia, flax):** Reduce inflammation, lower triglycerides, protect blood vessels.
- **Magnesium:** Relaxes blood vessels, improves insulin sensitivity, and supports heartbeat rhythm.
- **Meditation & stress reduction:** High stress = high cortisol = blood sugar + blood pressure spikes.
- **Walking after meals:** Improves blood flow, lowers glucose, reduces heart strain.
- **Regular movement:** Even light exercise daily improves circulation and keeps arteries flexible.

Key Takeaway

Complications don't have to be your story. By protecting nerves with B12 and ALA, shielding your eyes with lutein and bilberry, caring for your kidneys with hydration and nettle tea, and strengthening your heart with omega-3s and magnesium, you take back control.

The same steps that balance blood sugar also protect the most vulnerable parts of your body. Every meal, every walk, every breath is not just about avoiding a spike — it's about protecting your future health and independence.

Nighttime Blood Sugar & Dreams

For many people with blood sugar challenges, the night is when the body's secrets reveal themselves. Strange dreams, panic-like awakenings, vivid memories, and restless tossing often have less to do with the mind — and more to do with what the blood sugar is doing behind the scenes.

1. WHY BLOOD SUGAR SWINGS DISRUPT REM SLEEP

Sleep is not one steady state. We cycle through stages, including **REM (Rapid Eye Movement) sleep** — the stage of vivid dreams, memory processing, and emotional release.

- **Blood sugar crashes (hypoglycemia):** The brain suddenly runs low on fuel. It may trigger adrenaline to wake you up, often with a pounding heart, sweating, or strange dreams.
- **Blood sugar spikes (hyperglycemia):** High glucose makes it harder to enter deep, restorative sleep, and can cause frequent urination that disrupts the night.
- Both extremes pull you out of REM, leaving dreams fragmented and the brain unrested.

2. WHY SO MANY DIABETICS WAKE AT 3 AM

Many people notice a frustrating pattern: waking between **2–4 am.** There are two main reasons:

- **The "Liver Dump" (Somogyi Effect):** If your blood sugar dips too low, your liver releases stored glucose to rescue you. This rebound can wake you suddenly, sometimes with anxiety or a racing heart.
- **The Dawn Phenomenon:** In the early morning, cortisol and growth hormone naturally rise to prepare you for

waking. These hormones also raise blood sugar, sometimes spiking it before breakfast.

For someone with diabetes or insulin resistance, both events can feel like nightmares — literally.

3. DREAMS, MEMORY & THE SUGAR–BRAIN LINK

Your personal experiences of vivid, almost electric dreams during blood sugar crashes highlight something profound:

- The brain depends almost entirely on glucose at night.
- When supply wavers, neurons misfire → memories, emotions, and images flood consciousness in strange ways.
- This may explain why some people report panic attacks, hyperventilation, or even physical reactions tied to dreams when blood sugar drops.

In a sense, your brain is "dreaming for survival" — a cry for fuel.

4. BEDTIME RITUALS TO BALANCE BLOOD SUGAR

Food:

- Have a **light protein snack** before bed if you tend to crash (e.g., boiled egg, a spoon of nut butter, cottage cheese with cinnamon).
- Avoid heavy carb meals late at night — they spike and crash you while you sleep.

Teas & Herbs:

- **Chamomile or lavender tea** – calms the nervous system.
- **Cinnamon tea** – stabilizes glucose overnight.

- **Turmeric + ginger golden milk (unsweetened)** – reduces inflammation and supports sleep.

Relaxation Practices:

- **Reiki or meditation** before bed to calm stress hormones.
- **Breathwork (4-7-8 or box breathing):** Signals the body it's safe to rest.
- **Journaling or prayer:** Clears mental stress that could raise cortisol.

Lifestyle Tips:

- Keep a **regular bedtime** (the body thrives on rhythm).
- Limit screens in the hour before sleep (blue light disrupts melatonin).
- Keep water at your bedside — thirst can be an early sign of high sugar.

Key Takeaway
Your nights tell a story. Waking with panic, vivid dreams, or a racing heart is often not "just stress" — it's your blood sugar rhythm speaking. By stabilizing glucose before bed, supporting your nervous system, and listening to your dreams as signals, you can reclaim rest and restore the healing power of sleep.

Medications — What You Need to Know

For many people with diabetes, medication is part of the journey. Some feel relief when a doctor prescribes help. Others feel shame, fear, or frustration — as if taking medication means they "failed." Here's the truth: medications are **tools**, not verdicts. Used wisely, they can save lives and prevent complications. But like any tool, they come with benefits and side effects.

THE MAIN PLAYERS
Insulin

- **What it does:** Insulin is the hormone your body naturally makes to move sugar from the blood into cells. If your pancreas doesn't make enough (Type 1 or later-stage Type 2), injections may be needed.
- **Benefits:** Lifesaving, prevents dangerously high blood sugars, and protects organs from damage.
- **Side effects:** Weight gain, risk of low blood sugar if dosing isn't balanced with food and activity.
- **Key note:** Taking insulin doesn't mean you failed — it means your pancreas needs support.

Metformin

- **What it does:** Reduces the amount of sugar your liver releases into your bloodstream and makes cells more sensitive to insulin.
- **Benefits:** Often the first-line medication; inexpensive; helps protect the heart; may aid weight management.
- **Side effects:** Stomach upset, diarrhea, and sometimes B12 deficiency with long-term use.
- **Real-life tip:** Taking it with meals often reduces stomach issues.

SGLT2 Inhibitors (like Jardiance, Farxiga)

- **What they do:** Help your kidneys release excess sugar into the urine.
- **Benefits:** Lower blood sugar and blood pressure, protect the heart and kidneys.
- **Side effects:** More frequent urination, yeast infections, urinary tract infections, and dehydration risk.
- **Key note:** These drugs can be very protective for heart and kidney health, but require good hydration and hygiene.

GLP-1 Receptor Agonists (like Ozempic, Trulicity, Rybelsus)

- **What they do:** Mimic a natural hormone that slows digestion, increases insulin when you eat, and helps you feel fuller sooner.
- **Benefits:** Lower blood sugar, promote weight loss, reduce heart risk.
- **Side effects:** Nausea, vomiting, constipation, possible gallbladder issues, and rare risks of pancreatitis.
- **Key note:** These are powerful medications, but some people (like I experienced) may find the side effects outweigh the benefits.

BENEFITS VS. SIDE EFFECTS

Every medication is a balancing act:

- **Benefits:** Lower blood sugar, reduced complications, better energy, and organ protection.
- **Side effects:** Digestive upset, infections, hair loss, fatigue, or new symptoms.

What works well for one person may be miserable for another. That's why it's so important to **listen to your body and track your responses.**

WHEN TO PUSH FOR ADJUSTMENTS

Doctors often start with standard doses, but you have a right to advocate for changes if:

- Your blood sugar is still high despite taking the medication.
- Side effects are making your quality of life worse.
- You suspect interactions with other prescriptions.
- Your lifestyle changes (diet, movement, stress) may allow for lower doses.

Remember: medications are part of the toolbox, not the whole picture. Nutrition, stress management, movement, and spiritual health all matter just as much.

PERSONAL REFLECTION

I was given metformin, SGLT2 inhibitors, and later a GLP-1. Yes, they worked — but the side effects were intense: diarrhea, hair loss, constant trips to the bathroom. Each medication was a reminder that while drugs can help, they're not a free pass. I had to learn to balance both worlds: using medical tools while also working on lifestyle shifts to support my pancreas and my brain.

How Small Changes Can Reverse Symptoms

When you're facing diabetes, especially when you hear the words *Type 2* or *Type 3*, it can feel permanent and overwhelming. But research — and real people's stories — are proving that even **small lifestyle changes can reverse many symptoms.**

1. THE POWER OF SMALL ADJUSTMENTS

You don't have to overhaul your entire life in one dramatic step. The body responds beautifully to gradual, consistent changes:

- Swapping soda for water or herbal tea.
- Adding a 10–15 minute walk after meals.
- Building plates with more vegetables and fewer refined carbs.
- Going to bed 30 minutes earlier.

Each shift may feel tiny, but together they lower blood sugar, reduce inflammation, and ease stress on the pancreas and brain.

2. WHY THIS WORKS

Lifestyle RX and many forward-thinking clinicians emphasize that **Type 2 diabetes — and even the early stages of Type 3 (brain insulin resistance)** — are not life sentences. They are conditions of imbalance. By restoring balance, you give the body a chance to reset.

- **Blood sugar drops steadily.** Spikes smooth out, energy stabilizes.
- **Insulin sensitivity improves.** Muscles and brain cells start responding again.

- **The brain clears.** Fog lifts, mood stabilizes, memory improves.
- **Medication needs may lessen.** Under a doctor's supervision, many people reduce doses as balance returns.

3. THE MINDSET SHIFT

Instead of thinking, *"I have to give everything up,"* try:

- *"What one small thing can I change today?"*
- *"How can I bring more sweetness into my life that isn't food?"*
- *"What's the smallest habit I can stick with every day?"*

Consistency matters more than intensity. One sustainable change practiced daily is far more powerful than an unsustainable overhaul that fades after two weeks.

4. REALISTIC EXPECTATIONS

Reversal doesn't always mean "cure." It means reducing symptoms, restoring balance, and preventing complications. For some, blood sugar normalizes completely. For others, the gift is needing fewer medications, sleeping better, or protecting brain function for decades longer.

Why This Matters

The future of diabetes care is not just in stronger medications — it's in empowering people to use food, movement, rest, and mindfulness as medicine. Type 2 and Type 3 diabetes can often be **reversed or slowed** with these small, steady lifestyle shifts. The earlier you begin, the greater the impact — but it's *never too late* to create change.

LifestyleRx: A "Lifestyle Prescription" for Diabetes Reversal

LifestyleRx is a **virtual, physician-led program** designed to help people with **Type 2 diabetes or prediabetes** reverse or significantly improve their condition through lifestyle, not just medication.

Program Highlights:

- **100% Virtual & Accessible:** No in-person visits required—everything is done via video.
- **Physician-Led Guidance:** You'll work directly with a licensed doctor from your region, who collaborates with your primary care provider.
- **Group Sessions + Personal Visits:** The 12-week format includes weekly small group meetings led by physicians and individual consultations.

The 4+2 Reversal Strategy: What You'll Learn

LifestyleRx teaches the **4+2 Strategy** for reversing insulin resistance through focused, science-based lifestyle changes:

1. **Eat to Lower Insulin** – Whole-food, low glycemic meals rich in protein and fiber.
2. **Use Your Muscles** – Build up to 150–300 minutes of movement per week.
3. **Be Kind to Your Liver** – Reduce factors (like sugar, alcohol, and inflammation) that burden hepatic (liver) function.
4. **Restore Fat Burning** – Support losing stored fat through nutrition, timing, and activity.

+2: Address **stress** and **sleep**, which significantly influence insulin resistance.

Proven Outcomes & Accessibility

- **Impressive Success Rates:** Around **46% of participants reach A1C levels low enough to be considered in remission.**
- **High Patient Impact:** Among the 653 tracked patients—91% improved their A1C, and 44% brought it below 6.5%. Average reduction: 1.38%.
- **Insurance/Coverage:** In Canada (e.g., BC, AB, ON), the program is often covered through provincial healthcare or partners like LifeLabs.
- **U.S. Option:** Available with insurance coverage, making it accessible at little to no cost. Community Feedback: What People Are Saying

In forums like Reddit's r/prediabetes, participants shared varied experiences:

"I met with the LifestyleRx doctor ... I was told I have to lose 10 kg without mentioning how... The approach is not compassionate and seems cookie-cutter."

But others found better experiences:

"The doctor I had was very patient and took the time to explain his recommendations ... he instantly moulded his therapy plan to suit my situation."

These stories highlight the variability, emphasizing the importance of patient—doctor fit and self-advocacy within the program.

https://lifestylerx.io/

Summary: Is LifestyleRx Right for You?

Pros	Considerations
Virtual, physician-led, and structured for real results	Experiences may vary by provider; advocate for your needs
Based on proven reversal strategies	Not a quick fix—requires effort, honesty, and consistency
Often covered by insurance	Insurance coverage and provider match matter

When Life Throws You Curves

Managing blood sugar isn't about perfection — it's about resilience. Life is full of birthdays, vacations, restaurant meals, and unexpected stressors. Instead of seeing these moments as failures, think of them as practice runs for living well with flexibility.

TRAVEL & EATING OUT

- **Plan Ahead, Don't Obsess:** Look at menus before you go. Identify meals with protein + veggies + healthy fats.
- **Snacks for the Road:** Pack nuts, jerky, or protein bars so you're not stuck with only fast food.
- **Airports & Hotels:** Walk the terminals, choose grilled over fried, ask for veggies instead of fries.
- **Hydration is Key:** Long trips = dehydration, which spikes blood sugar. Keep water handy.

HOLIDAYS & CELEBRATIONS

- **Pick Your Favorites:** Instead of a little of everything, choose the one or two treats you *really* love.
- **Anchor the Plate:** Fill half your plate with veggies and protein before adding starchy sides.
- **Slow Down:** Eating slowly helps your body manage sugar more evenly.
- **Walk It Off:** A 10–15 minute stroll after a holiday meal is one of the best gifts you can give your pancreas.

DEALING WITH CRAVINGS & STRESS

Cravings are not weakness — they're chemistry. High stress, poor sleep, or recent sugar spikes can all drive "urgent hunger."

Tools to Help:

- **The 20-Minute Rule:** Cravings often pass if you give yourself 20 minutes with water, tea, or a short walk.
- **Protein First:** If you're craving sugar, try a boiled egg, string cheese, or a handful of nuts. A stabilizing protein often quiets the craving.
- **Stress Reset:** Deep breathing, a quick journal entry, or stepping outside can break the cortisol-sugar craving loop.

UNEXPECTED SPIKES

Sometimes, even with your best effort, blood sugar will run high. Instead of panic:

- **Hydrate:** Water helps flush excess sugar.
- **Move:** A brisk 10-minute walk can lower sugar as effectively as medication in some cases.
- **Reflect, Don't Judge:** Ask, "What triggered this?" A missed meal? Hidden carbs? Stress? This builds awareness instead of guilt.

HOW TO RECOVER AFTER A SETBACK

We all slip — and that's okay. What matters most is the next step, not the stumble.

1. **Forgive Yourself:** Guilt raises stress, which raises blood sugar.
2. **Reset the Next Meal:** Don't starve yourself — just go back to protein + veggies + healthy fat.

3. **Learn & Adjust:** Every setback is feedback. What can you do differently next time?
4. **Keep the Long View:** One spike won't ruin your progress, but a habit of giving up will.

PERSONAL REFLECTION

I've been "that person" at the holiday table, both giving in to cravings and feeling ashamed afterward. I've woken in the night panicked after a day of poor choices. What I've learned is this: diabetes management is not about never falling, but about learning to stand up faster each time.

REFLECTION PROMPTS

- What situations trigger you to eat or drink differently (holidays, stress, travel)?
- When you wake at night, how do you usually respond — with panic, food, prayer, or breathing?
- What bedtime ritual helps you feel calm and safe?

Emotional + Spiritual Healing: The Sweetness Beyond Sugar

CRAVINGS OF THE BODY VS. CRAVINGS OF THE SOUL

Sugar cravings can feel overpowering, as if your body is moving on its own. But sometimes what you're really craving isn't food at all. It's comfort. Rest. Connection. Joy.

The body calls for "sweetness," and the quickest delivery system is sugar. But your soul knows that true sweetness is found elsewhere. When you slow down and ask, *"What am I really hungry for?"* the answer is often: love, peace, laughter, or meaning.

FINDING SWEETNESS WITHOUT SUGAR

- **Connection:** Call a friend, hug your partner, play with your pet. Love balances blood sugar better than candy.
- **Rest:** Sometimes exhaustion disguises itself as hunger. A nap or quiet breath may satisfy more than a snack.
- **Creativity:** Painting, music, writing, gardening — these bring joy without a sugar crash.
- **Spiritual Nourishment:** Prayer, meditation, gratitude, or sitting in nature can fill the deep hunger for peace and belonging.
- **Pleasure:** A bath, warm blanket, fresh flowers, candlelight — sweetness for the senses.

HEALING EMOTIONS STORED IN SUGAR

Many people with diabetes or sugar struggles also carry emotional wounds: grief, disappointment, loneliness, or unfulfilled dreams. Sugar provides a quick but false comfort.

Real healing begins when you allow yourself to feel, release, and soften into those emotions instead of numbing them.

Tools for Emotional Release:

- **Journaling:** "When I crave sugar, what am I really craving?"
- **Breathwork:** Inhale peace, exhale fear.
- **Energy Work:** Reiki or reflexology to release stored tension.
- **Affirmations:** *"I replace sugar with the sweetness of spirit, connection, and gratitude."*

THE SWEETNESS OF LIFE PRACTICE

Each day, give yourself one act of true sweetness:

- A slow walk in the sun.
- A moment of prayer or stillness.
- Laughter with someone you love.
- Writing down one thing that brings you joy.

Over time, these practices re-train the brain: sweetness is not in the cupboard — it's in your life.

Balancing blood sugar is not only about food or medication — it is about restoring **joy, love, and meaning.** When you nourish the soul, cravings loosen their grip, and healing becomes not just about managing disease, but about reclaiming life's deepest sweetness.

Prevention for the Next Generation

If I could go back and talk to my 18-year-old self, I would tell her that those shaky hands, sugar crashes, and headaches weren't just "quirks." They were early warning signs. I would tell her that prevention is possible, that small choices made young can change the entire course of a life.

LESSONS I WISH I KNEW AT 18

- **Sugar Highs Aren't Harmless:** That one drink that knocked me out, those cravings that felt unstoppable — they were my body waving a red flag.
- **Carbs Are Not All the Same:** White bread, soda, and pasta don't fuel the brain — they confuse it. Fiber-rich carbs keep energy steady.
- **Sleep & Stress Matter:** Those late nights studying or worrying weren't just tiring me out, they were spiking my blood sugar.
- **Movement Isn't About Weight:** Exercise is a way to keep your cells open to insulin — even if the scale doesn't move.

WHAT PARENTS SHOULD WATCH FOR

Blood sugar imbalance often starts decades before a diabetes diagnosis. Warning signs in children and teens can include:

- Constant hunger, especially for sweets or refined carbs.
- Irritability or "hanger" between meals.
- Difficulty concentrating or frequent brain fog.
- Sudden crashes in energy (especially mid-morning or mid-afternoon).
- Weight gain around the belly, even with average eating.

For middle-aged adults, watch for:

- Blurry vision, especially after eating.
- Nighttime sweats, panic, or strange dreams.
- Needing caffeine and sugar to "get through the day."
- Mixing up words, forgetting why you walked into a room.
- Slow healing cuts or frequent infections.

These signs don't mean someone *has* diabetes, but they are signals worth checking.

HOPE: DIABETES DOESN'T HAVE TO BECOME DEMENTIA

The term **"Type 3 diabetes"** was coined because scientists saw a link between insulin resistance and Alzheimer's disease. But this is not a sentence — it's a warning, and a chance for prevention.

Studies show that:

- People who stabilize their blood sugar cut their dementia risk significantly.
- Movement, good sleep, and balanced meals protect the brain as much as they protect the pancreas.
- Even those with diabetes for decades can still slow or prevent brain decline by taking action now.

THE GENERATIONAL GIFT

If you're reading this, you have the chance to give your children, grandchildren, or students a better path. Talk openly about food, cravings, stress, and energy — not just weight. Model balance rather than restriction. Share the truth that health is about how we feel and function, not just how we look.

The next generation can learn what we didn't know. They can live free of the cycle of spikes, crashes, medications, and fear. Prevention isn't perfect, but every step matters.

Part V – A Path Forward

Your Blood Sugar Reset Plan

Knowledge is power — but only if it's put into action. This 30-day plan is not about perfection or punishment. It's about giving your body and brain a reset: steadier energy, calmer moods, clearer thinking, and lower blood sugar swings.

Think of it as a **trial run** for a new way of living. By the end of the month, you'll know what works for *you* and what habits you want to carry forward.

THE FOUR PILLARS OF THE RESET

1. **Food — Balanced & Steady**
   - Follow the **50/25/25 Method** ("How Much" aspect):
     - 50% veggies
     - 25% protein
     - 25% smart carbs + drizzle of healthy fat
   - Crowd out cravings with nutrient-dense meals instead of trying to "white-knuckle" willpower.
   - Limit added sugar and refined carbs — allow 3 days for cravings to pass.
2. **Movement — Daily Energy Use**
   - Aim for **10–15 minutes of walking each day,** *and if possible,* **after each meal.**
   - Add 2–3 sessions a week of strength or resistance training to open up muscle "glucose doors."

TYPE 3 DIABETES | 143

- o   Keep it gentle if needed — walking and stretching count.
3. **Stress & Sleep — Reset Your Hormones**
   - o   Practice **2 - 5 minutes of deep breathing** or meditation daily.
   - o   Keep a bedtime routine — aim for 7–8 hours of sleep.
   - o   Journal before bed to calm your brain.
4. **Self-Tracking — Know Your Patterns**
   - o   Track meals, moods, and energy in a simple journal.
   - o   Optional: use a glucometer or continuous glucose monitor (if accessible) to see real-time feedback.

Understanding Cravings: Why They Hit Hard

When you cut out fast carbs (sweets, bread, rice, potatoes, pasta), your body goes through a mini "withdrawal." Here's why:

- **Dopamine & Reward Pathways:** Sugar lights up the brain's reward centers, like a drug. When you stop, the brain panics and says, *"Where's my quick hit?"*
- **Blood Sugar Swings:** If you've been eating fast carbs, your body is used to sharp rises and falls. Taking them away feels like a drop-off at first.
- **Gut Microbiome Influence:** Certain gut bacteria thrive on sugar and actually send signals (via cravings) to push you to feed them. When you starve them, they protest — loudly.
- **Habit Loops:** Often, cravings are tied to routines (dessert after dinner, afternoon snack at work). Breaking the pattern feels uncomfortable, even if you're not hungry.

The good news? After about **3 days** of low or no fast carbs, cravings usually quieten because blood sugar stabilizes, dopamine receptors reset, and your body remembers how to burn fat for energy.

3-Day "Craving Survival Diet"

The goal here is **not deprivation** — it's to *stabilize blood sugar fast* so cravings fade.

Day 1 — Stabilization Start

- **Breakfast:** 2 boiled eggs + sautéed spinach in olive oil + half an avocado.
- **Snack:** A handful of almonds or walnuts.
- **Lunch:** Grilled chicken breast + large salad (mixed greens, cucumbers, peppers, olive oil + lemon).
- **Snack:** Celery sticks with almond butter.
- **Dinner:** Salmon or trout + roasted broccoli + cauliflower mash (instead of potatoes).
- **Evening craving rescue:** Cinnamon tea or warm turmeric latte (unsweetened).

Day 2 — Ride Out the Dip

(Cravings often feel strongest this day — stay busy, hydrate, and keep snacks handy.)

- **Breakfast:** Greek yogurt (unsweetened, full-fat) + chia seeds + a few berries.
- **Snack:** Cheese stick + cucumber slices.
- **Lunch:** Turkey burger (no bun) with sautéed zucchini + side salad.
- **Snack:** Handful of pumpkin seeds.
- **Dinner:** Stir-fry with chicken or tofu, broccoli, cabbage, garlic, and ginger. Serve over cauliflower rice.
- **Evening craving rescue:** Herbal tea with a splash of coconut milk.

Day 3 — Breaking Through

(Cravings usually ease here — energy feels steadier.)

- **Breakfast:** Scrambled eggs with mushrooms + avocado slices.
- **Snack:** A few Brazil nuts or sunflower seeds.
- **Lunch:** Grilled shrimp or chicken Caesar salad (no croutons, light on dressing).
- **Snack:** Half an avocado with sea salt and lime.
- **Dinner:** Baked chicken thighs + roasted Brussels sprouts + spaghetti squash.
- **Evening craving rescue:** Rooibos tea or ginger tea.

TIPS TO GET THROUGH THE 3-DAY CRAVING RESET

Cutting out fast carbs and sweets is not just about food — it's about retraining your **brain, body, and habits** all at once. These tips help soften the process, so you don't feel like you're battling yourself every hour.

1. HYDRATION = KEY

Many cravings are actually mild dehydration in disguise. When you're thirsty, your body sometimes signals it as "hunger," especially for something quick like sugar.

- Start each morning with a full glass of water.
- Keep herbal teas handy — cinnamon, peppermint, ginger, or rooibos can "scratch the itch" for flavor without sugar.
- Add lemon, cucumber, or mint to water for variety.
- Rule of thumb: before giving in to a craving, drink a glass of water and wait 10 minutes.

2. PROTEIN AT EVERY MEAL

Protein is your anchor food. It digests slowly, keeps you full, and prevents the "urgent hunger" that sends you searching for cookies.

- Aim for at least **20–30 grams per meal** (e.g., 2 eggs + Greek yogurt, or a chicken breast + beans).
- Snacks count too: a cheese stick, boiled egg, or handful of nuts beats a granola bar any day.
- Think of protein as a "shield" against sugar cravings — it quiets the rollercoaster.

3. CINNAMON, VANILLA, OR MINT — SWEET TRICKS WITHOUT SUGAR

Your brain craves sweetness partly out of habit. Certain flavors can "trick" it into satisfaction without actual sugar.

- **Cinnamon:** Add to tea, coffee, or sprinkle on plain yogurt. Balances blood sugar while tasting sweet.
- **Vanilla extract:** A drop in tea or warm milk mimics a dessert.
- **Mint:** Fresh mint leaves, peppermint tea, or even sugar-free mint gum can cool the craving cycle.
  These flavors remind the brain of sweetness while actually calming it.

4. MOVEMENT — YOUR SECRET WEAPON

When a craving feels unbearable, move your body.

- A **10-minute brisk walk** lowers stress hormones and helps muscles pull sugar out of your bloodstream.
- Even pacing around the house, stretching, or a few squats works.

- Movement doesn't just burn calories — it stabilizes blood sugar and distracts the brain from the craving spiral.

5. PERMISSION TO EAT

This isn't about starvation. When you're genuinely hungry, eat — just eat the right foods.

- Protein + healthy fats + fiber-rich veggies = a satisfied brain and belly.
- Examples: boiled eggs with avocado, chicken with broccoli, nuts with cheese.
- Starving yourself backfires, making the next craving stronger.

THE BREAKTHROUGH AFTER DAY 3

The first 72 hours are the toughest — but on the other side is relief:

- **Brain fog lifts.** Your thoughts feel sharper, words come easier.
- **Energy steadies.** No more highs and crashes — you start to feel level.
- **Cravings shrink.** They don't disappear forever, but they lose their "urgency."
- **Mood improves.** Less irritability, less of that panicky "hangry" feeling.

From here, you can reintroduce **slow, fiber-rich carbs** if you choose:

- Quinoa
- Lentils & beans
- Oats
- Sweet potatoes in small portions

These foods release sugar slowly, unlike bread, soda, or candy, so they fuel without the crash.

Key Takeaway: Think of these 3 days as a bridge — from being controlled by cravings to being in control of cravings. Once you cross it, the freedom you feel will motivate you to keep going.

Breakfast:

BEST TIME TO EAT BREAKFAST (AND INTERMITTENT FASTING CONSIDERATIONS)

Type 1 Diabetes

- **Breakfast timing:** Important to eat within 1–2 hours of waking, because insulin dosing and blood sugar monitoring are tightly linked. Skipping breakfast can increase the risk of hypoglycemia (especially if insulin was taken earlier) or later spikes.
- **Focus:** A *low-glycemic, protein-rich breakfast* is best (e.g., eggs + avocado + veggies, or Greek yogurt with nuts).
- **Fasting caution:** Intermittent fasting is **not typically recommended** without very close medical supervision, since insulin therapy must be carefully matched to food timing.

Type 2 Diabetes

- **Breakfast timing:** Eating within the first **2–3 hours after waking** helps prevent mid-morning blood sugar crashes. Skipping breakfast can sometimes cause higher blood sugar later in the day (the "second meal effect"), especially if lunch ends up being carb-heavy.
- **Best practice:** Start with **protein + fiber + healthy fat** to keep glucose stable the rest of the day.
- **Intermittent fasting:** Some people with Type 2 benefit from a **16:8 fasting schedule** (first meal at 10–11 AM, last meal by 6–7 PM). Research shows it may improve insulin sensitivity and weight loss, but only if meals are balanced (not high-carb). Blood sugar monitoring is essential to make sure fasting doesn't cause spikes or dips.

Type 3 Diabetes (Insulin Resistance in the Brain / Alzheimer's link)

- **Breakfast timing:** Early eating seems protective for the brain. A **protein-rich meal within 1–2 hours of waking** helps regulate neurotransmitters and reduces brain fog/cravings.
- **Why:** Skipping breakfast in insulin-resistant individuals often worsens cravings, mood swings, and mental fatigue later in the day.
- **Fasting caution:** Intermittent fasting can be helpful **if it feels good for the brain** (e.g., a 12–14 hour overnight fast, like stopping eating at 7 PM and breakfast at 9 AM). But long fasts (16+ hours) may backfire, leading to hypoglycemia, fatigue, or more carb cravings once eating begins.

THE ROLE OF CORTISOL & BLOOD SUGAR IN THE MORNING

- Cortisol naturally spikes in the early morning (the "dawn phenomenon"), which raises blood sugar slightly.
- Eating a balanced breakfast (protein + fat + fiber) *anchors* blood sugar and keeps it from rising too much.
- Skipping breakfast can exaggerate this spike, especially in Type 2 and Type 3 diabetics.

PRACTICAL GUIDELINES

- **Type 1:** Breakfast within 1–2 hours, always with medical supervision for insulin dosing.
- **Type 2:** Flexible — within 2–3 hours of waking, or late-morning if doing gentle intermittent fasting. Always pair carbs with protein/fat.
- **Type 3:** Earlier is better — protein in the morning supports brain health and reduces cognitive dips.

RULE OF THUMB FOR ALL TYPES:

- Never break a fast with *pure carbs* (fruit, cereal, toast, etc.). Always start with **protein first** to blunt the blood sugar rise.
- If experimenting with fasting, track how you *feel* (energy, cravings, clarity) and, if possible, measure glucose levels to see how your body responds.

30 Blood Sugar–Friendly Breakfasts

EGG-BASED (PROTEIN ANCHORS)

1. Scrambled eggs with spinach + avocado
2. Omelet with mushrooms, peppers, and feta cheese
3. Poached eggs over sautéed kale with olive oil
4. Hard-boiled eggs with cucumber slices and hummus
5. Egg muffins (baked eggs with veggies + turkey or chicken sausage)

YOGURT & SMOOTHIE OPTIONS (WATCH THE SUGAR!)

6. Full-fat Greek yogurt + chia seeds + handful of berries
7. Cottage cheese bowl with walnuts + cinnamon + sliced apple
8. Smoothie: unsweetened almond milk, spinach, avocado, protein powder, and a few blueberries
9. Chia seed pudding (made with unsweetened almond milk, cinnamon, and topped with nuts)
10. Kefir (unsweetened) with ground flaxseed and pumpkin seeds

HIGH-PROTEIN, LOW-CARB ALTERNATIVES

11. Turkey bacon with scrambled eggs and tomatoes
12. Smoked salmon with cream cheese + cucumber slices (skip the bagel)
13. Leftover grilled chicken breast with sautéed veggies (breakfast doesn't have to be "breakfast food")
14. Turkey or chicken sausage with roasted Brussels sprouts
15. Shakshuka (eggs poached in spiced tomato + pepper sauce)

FIBER-RICH CARBS (SLOW RELEASE)

16. Steel-cut oats topped with walnuts, chia seeds, and cinnamon (skip brown sugar/honey)
17. Overnight oats with almond butter + flaxseed + a sprinkle of berries
18. Quinoa breakfast bowl with almond milk, pumpkin seeds, and unsweetened coconut flakes
19. Sweet potato hash with spinach + fried egg on top
20. Buckwheat pancakes (small portion, topped with nut butter instead of syrup)

QUICK & ON-THE-GO OPTIONS

21. Protein shake (unsweetened protein powder, almond milk, spinach, flaxseed)
22. Handful of nuts + string cheese + hard-boiled egg
23. Low-carb wrap filled with scrambled eggs + avocado
24. Apple slices with almond butter + sprinkle of cinnamon
25. Jerky (low-sugar) + handful of walnuts + cucumber sticks

PLANT-BASED & VEGAN-FRIENDLY

26. Tofu scramble with peppers + nutritional yeast
27. Lentil patties with avocado slices
28. Chia + flax porridge (instead of oatmeal) with almond butter
29. Green smoothie (unsweetened almond milk, kale, hemp seeds, avocado, cinnamon)
30. Vegan yogurt (unsweetened coconut or almond) with pumpkin seeds + blueberries

PRO TIPS FOR BREAKFAST SUCCESS

- **Avoid naked carbs.** Never eat fruit, oats, or bread alone — always pair with protein or fat.
- **Make it savory, not sweet.** A savory breakfast keeps cravings away better than a sweet one.
- **Think leftovers.** Dinner foods (chicken, fish, veggies) make excellent breakfasts.
- **Batch prep.** Make egg muffins, chia pudding, or overnight oats in advance for grab-and-go.

With this list, you've got a **30-day breakfast rotation** that stabilizes blood sugar, avoids spikes, and still feels varied and satisfying.

Lunch:

Best Time to Eat Lunch (and Pre-Lunch Snacks)

GENERAL RULE OF THUMB

- Aim for lunch **4–5 hours after breakfast.**
- The goal is to **avoid both extremes**: long fasting that leads to crashes OR grazing that keeps insulin elevated all day.
- Think of lunch as your *anchor meal* that carries you through the afternoon (a danger zone for cravings and fatigue).

TYPE 1 DIABETES

- **Timing:** Lunch should be consistent day-to-day because insulin dosing depends on predictability. Waiting too long risks hypoglycemia (if insulin was taken for breakfast) or post-lunch spikes (if too hungry and eating too fast).
- **Best window:** Around **midday (11:30 AM–1:00 PM)**, depending on breakfast timing.
- **Pre-lunch snacks:** Sometimes necessary if blood sugar dips. Good options: a boiled egg, a cheese stick, or a small handful of nuts. Avoid fruit or crackers alone (spikes too fast).

TYPE 2 DIABETES

- **Timing:** Consistency matters less than balance. Most do well with lunch around **12:00–1:30 PM**, ~4–5 hours after breakfast.
- **If breakfast was small or skipped:** A balanced snack mid-morning can prevent the "hangry crash" at lunch (which usually leads to overeating).
  - o Snack examples:
    - Celery + almond butter
    - Handful of nuts + cheese
    - Half an avocado with sea salt
  - o Avoid carb-only snacks (granola bars, fruit juice).
- **If breakfast was hearty:** You may not need a snack at all — going straight to lunch is fine.

TYPE 3 DIABETES (SUGAR–BRAIN CONNECTION)

- **Timing:** Eating every **3–4 hours** can prevent brain fog, word mix-ups, and memory lapses caused by dips in glucose delivery to brain cells. Lunch should not be delayed.
- **Best window: 12:00–12:30 PM** if breakfast was at 8:00–9:00 AM.
- **Pre-lunch snacks:** Helpful if brain fog or cravings strike before lunch.
  - o Examples:
    - Greek yogurt with chia seeds
    - A handful of walnuts or sunflower seeds
    - A boiled egg + cucumber slices
  - o The goal is *brain fuel without a spike*.

PRACTICAL TIPS FOR ALL TYPES

- **Listen to signals:** Shakiness, sudden hunger, irritability, or brain fog before lunch = your body is asking for stabilization. Don't ignore it.
- **Protein + fat in snacks:** These quiet cravings help prevent sharp insulin spikes.
- **Watch the clock:** Skipping lunch or eating it late often backfires with afternoon sugar spikes and nighttime episodes.

Key Takeaway:

- **Type 1:** Lunch timing is tied to insulin, consistency is crucial. Snacks may be needed.
- **Type 2:** Lunch ~4–5 hours after breakfast. Snack only if breakfast was small/skipped.
- **Type 3:** Lunch on time (not late), snack if brain fog or cravings appear.

Mixing Breakfast and Lunch

(10–11 AM Meal)

Why It Works for Some

- Eating later can help keep insulin levels lower in the morning (when cortisol is already naturally high).
- A bigger, balanced meal at 10–11 AM can provide enough fuel to carry you through the afternoon without crashes.
- It may reduce the total number of blood sugar "spikes" in the day, which is especially helpful for insulin resistance.

TYPE 1 DIABETES

- **Caution:** Timing meals later can be tricky because insulin dosing is based on expected food intake.
- If skipping breakfast, close monitoring is essential to prevent hypoglycemia from morning insulin or activity.
- A **10–11 AM "brunch"** should be hearty: protein + fat + some slow carbs.
  - Example: Omelet with veggies + avocado + side of lentils or quinoa.
- Best done **only if coordinated with the insulin plan**.

TYPE 2 DIABETES

- **Benefit:** Many people with Type 2 find that pushing the first meal to 10–11 AM (intermittent fasting style, 16:8) improves insulin sensitivity, lowers fasting glucose, and aids weight loss.
- The key is making the **brunch meal balanced and filling,** not carb-heavy.
  - Example: Grilled chicken salad with avocado + a boiled egg OR scrambled eggs with spinach and roasted sweet potato.
- Often, this schedule looks like:
  - **10:30 AM brunch**
  - **3:30–4 PM snack (protein + fat)**
  - **6:30–7 PM dinner**

TYPE 3 DIABETES (SUGAR–BRAIN CONNECTION)

- **Consideration:** For the brain, long fasting may backfire — some people feel more foggy or anxious if they go too long without fuel.
- A **10–11 AM meal can work,** but only if:
  - You hydrate and maybe have **a light stabilizer early morning** (like green tea + a few nuts, or half an avocado).

○ The 10–11 AM meal is **protein-rich** to stabilize brain glucose delivery.

○ Example: Salmon + spinach + avocado bowl OR Greek yogurt with seeds, nuts, and berries.

PRO TIPS FOR A 10–11 AM BRUNCH MEAL

- **Make it bigger than breakfast, lighter than dinner.** Enough protein and fat to carry you 4–5 hours.
- **Avoid carb-only meals** (like pancakes, toast, fruit bowls) — these will crash you by mid-afternoon.
- **Plan a light afternoon "bridge snack"** (nuts, cheese, boiled egg, veggie sticks + hummus) so you don't arrive at dinner overly hungry.
- **Hydrate in the morning** (water, tea, coffee without sugar) so dehydration doesn't disguise itself as hunger.

KEY TAKEAWAY:

- **Type 1:** Possible, but requires insulin adjustment.
- **Type 2:** Often very beneficial if the meal is balanced.
- **Type 3:** Can work, but may need a small stabilizer earlier to avoid brain fog.

The Second Meal Effect

The "second meal effect" is the idea that **what and when you eat at one meal influences your blood sugar response at the** *next* **meal.**

HOW IT WORKS

- When you eat a balanced meal (protein, healthy fat, and fiber), your blood sugar rises slowly and your body releases insulin more effectively.
- That meal "primes" your metabolism for the next one — your body becomes better at handling the glucose from the following meal.
- On the flip side, if you skip breakfast or eat a carb-heavy meal (like cereal, toast, or a muffin), your blood sugar spikes quickly and crashes. That sets you up for worse spikes and crashes later in the day.

Example

- **Scenario A (balanced breakfast):**
  - o Breakfast: Omelet with spinach + avocado
  - o Lunch: Even if you eat something with carbs (like quinoa salad), your blood sugar doesn't spike as much, because your morning protein/fiber "trained" your body to handle glucose better.
- **Scenario B (skipped breakfast):**
  - o No food until lunch.
  - o Lunch: Same quinoa salad as above, but now your blood sugar spikes higher because your body wasn't "primed" earlier.

WHY IT MATTERS FOR DIABETICS

- **Type 1:** Meal timing and balance are critical for insulin dosing. Skipping meals can cause unpredictable highs/lows.
- **Type 2:** The second meal effect is especially powerful. Studies show that eating a low-carb, high-protein breakfast can cut after-lunch blood sugar spikes by **up to 30–40%.**
- **Type 3 (brain-related insulin resistance):** Balanced meals help reduce brain fog and cognitive dips throughout the day. If you skip or eat a high-carb breakfast, you may notice worse mood swings and memory issues later.

KEY TRICKS TO HARNESS THE SECOND MEAL EFFECT

1. **Never skip breakfast** (unless you're intentionally fasting *and* your blood sugar handles it well).
2. **Protein first:** Eating protein at the start of a meal slows digestion and reduces glucose spikes.
3. **Vinegar hack:** Having 1–2 tsp of apple cider vinegar in water before a meal can blunt the spike of the next meal.
4. **Veggies before carbs:** Eating a salad or non-starchy vegetables first lowers the glucose impact of whatever comes after.
5. **Evening matters:** A balanced dinner helps regulate fasting glucose levels the next morning.

Key Takeaway: Every meal is connected. Think of your meals like a chain reaction — one sets the tone for the next. By "front-loading" your day with protein and fiber, you make your metabolism and brain more resilient for the meals that follow.

30 Blood Sugar–Friendly Lunches

SALAD POWER BOWLS

1. Grilled chicken salad with mixed greens, cucumber, peppers, olive oil + lemon
2. Salmon salad with spinach, avocado, and pumpkin seeds
3. Greek salad (feta, olives, cucumber, tomato) + grilled chicken
4. Cobb salad with turkey, avocado, hard-boiled eggs, and olive oil dressing
5. Taco salad (ground turkey, lettuce, salsa, avocado, black beans)

LOW-CARB WRAPS & BOWLS

6. Turkey and avocado lettuce wraps
7. Egg salad or tuna salad lettuce wraps
8. Chicken Caesar salad wrap in a low-carb tortilla or collard greens
9. Shrimp & avocado bowl with cauliflower rice
10. Turkey burger "bowl" with sautéed zucchini and mushrooms

WARM PROTEIN + VEGGIE PLATES

11. Grilled salmon with roasted Brussels sprouts and side salad
12. Baked chicken thighs with broccoli and cauliflower mash
13. Turkey meatballs with spaghetti squash and marinara
14. Beef stir-fry with broccoli, peppers, and garlic (served over cauliflower rice)
15. Grilled pork chops with green beans and salad

VEGETARIAN / PLANT-BASED OPTIONS

16. Lentil soup with kale and olive oil drizzle
17. Quinoa + roasted veggie bowl (add chickpeas or tofu)
18. Black bean chili with avocado garnish
19. Greek yogurt + flaxseed + walnuts + side of cucumber and tomato
20. Tofu stir-fry with bok choy, garlic, and sesame seeds

MEAL PREP FRIENDLY

21. Grilled chicken breast + roasted veggie medley (carrots, zucchini, peppers)
22. Hard-boiled eggs + mixed greens + avocado
23. Leftover roasted salmon turned into a salad with olive oil + lemon
24. Deli turkey roll-ups with cream cheese and cucumber slices
25. Mason jar salad (layered greens, protein, veggies, seeds, dressing at the bottom)

QUICK & ON-THE-GO

26. Tuna pouch with avocado + baby carrots
27. Hummus + veggie sticks + boiled egg
28. Cottage cheese + cherry tomatoes + sunflower seeds
29. Leftover grilled steak strips + spinach salad
30. Chicken soup with extra veggies and olive oil drizzle

PRO TIPS FOR LUNCH SUCCESS

- **Always anchor with protein** (chicken, fish, tofu, beans, or eggs).
- **Use leftovers** from dinner to save time — reheated protein + fresh greens = instant lunch.
- **Keep emergency snacks** (nuts, seeds, tuna pouch) for days you don't have time.

- **Avoid naked carbs.** If you want a small portion of quinoa, beans, or sweet potato, *always pair it with protein and fat.*

With this 30-day list, you've got a **full month of steady-energy lunches** that can be mixed, matched, and meal-prepped.

When & If Snacks Are Needed

TYPE 1 DIABETES

- **When:** Snacks may be essential, especially if there's a risk of hypoglycemia between meals or overnight.
- **Best practice:** Pair **protein + fat** with any carb if needed. Example: apple + cheese, not apple alone.
- **Night snacks:** Sometimes needed to prevent overnight lows — something with protein (like Greek yogurt with chia).

TYPE 2 DIABETES

- **When:** If meals are **balanced and filling**, snacks may not be necessary. However, they can be helpful if:
  - o Breakfast or lunch was small/light.
  - o Blood sugar is dipping (shakiness, irritability, urgent hunger).
- **Best practice:** Use snacks strategically, not out of habit. Focus on protein/fat/fiber — not "quick carbs."

TYPE 3 DIABETES (SUGAR–BRAIN CONNECTION)

- **When:** The brain needs a steady stream of glucose, so skipping meals or long gaps may worsen brain fog, word mix-ups, or mood swings. A **mid-morning or mid-afternoon snack** can help stabilize.
- **Best practice:** Small, nutrient-dense snacks with protein/fat. Avoid sugar-only options (which cause brain crashes).

30 Blood Sugar–Friendly Snacks

PROTEIN + FAT ANCHORS

1. Hard-boiled egg + cucumber slices
2. Cheese stick + cherry tomatoes
3. Deli turkey roll-ups (turkey + avocado slices wrapped in lettuce)
4. Greek yogurt (unsweetened, full-fat) + cinnamon
5. Cottage cheese + sliced cucumber or radish
6. Beef jerky (low-sugar) + handful of walnuts
7. Tuna pouch + celery sticks
8. Smoked salmon roll-ups with cream cheese

NUTS & SEEDS (PORTABLE OPTIONS)

9. Almonds + 85% dark chocolate square
10. Walnuts + blueberries (small handful)
11. Sunflower seeds + string cheese
12. Pumpkin seeds + cucumber slices
13. Brazil nuts + hard-boiled egg
14. Flax crackers + avocado mash
15. Chia seed pudding (unsweetened, small portion)

VEGGIE-BASED SNACKS

16. Baby carrots + hummus
17. Bell pepper strips + guacamole
18. Celery sticks + almond butter
19. Roasted edamame or chickpeas (lightly seasoned)
20. Zucchini chips baked with olive oil

FRUIT + PROTEIN/FAT PAIRINGS

21. Apple slices + almond butter
22. Pear slices + goat cheese
23. Berries + whipped coconut cream (unsweetened)
24. Banana (½) + peanut butter (if tolerated well, small portion)
25. Grapes + string cheese (small handful of grapes)

QUICK & COMFORTING

26. Deviled eggs with avocado filling
27. Turkey or chicken meatballs (make ahead, keep chilled)
28. Mini protein smoothie (unsweetened almond milk, protein powder, spinach)
29. Leftover roasted chicken strips + cucumber slices
30. Warm turmeric or cinnamon latte + handful of nuts

TIMING SNACK STRATEGIES

- **Morning snack (10–11 AM):** Best if breakfast was light or delayed. Choose protein + fat to avoid a spike.
- **Afternoon snack (3–4 PM):** Prevents the "crash" before dinner. Helpful especially for Type 3 (brain fog).
- **Evening snack (7–8 PM):** Sometimes needed for Type 1 or if dinner was early/light. Stick to protein + fat to prevent overnight crashes.

KEY TAKEAWAY:

- **Type 1:** Snacks may be necessary, especially for safety.
- **Type 2:** Optional — use them as tools, not habits.
- **Type 3:** Often beneficial for brain steadiness.

Snack Survival Guide

When Snacks Help Most

Time of Day	Type 1	Type 2	Type 3 (Brain Connection)
Mid-Morning (10–11 AM)	Helpful if breakfast was light or insulin taken earlier	Only if breakfast was small or skipped	Often helpful to prevent brain fog or word mix-ups
Afternoon (3–4 PM)	May be needed if lunch insulin was strong	Useful if lunch was light or cravings strike	Recommended — stabilizes brain before dinner
Evening (7–8 PM)	Sometimes necessary to prevent overnight lows	Usually not needed unless dinner was early/light	May help reduce nighttime episodes or panic awakenings

SNACK TYPES BY GOAL
Steady Blood Sugar (Protein + Fat)

- Boiled egg + cucumber slices
- Cheese stick + cherry tomatoes
- Deli turkey roll-ups with avocado
- Handful of nuts (almonds, walnuts, Brazil nuts)
- Cottage cheese + sliced cucumber

Brain Fuel (Protein + Fiber)

- Greek yogurt (unsweetened) + chia seeds
- Apple slices + almond butter
- Berries + handful of walnuts
- Tuna pouch + celery sticks
- Chia pudding (unsweetened, small portion)

Comfort Snacks (Warm & Craving-Busting)

- Cinnamon tea with roasted pumpkin seeds
- Warm turmeric latte + handful of sunflower seeds
- Deviled eggs (with avocado or Greek yogurt filling)
- Roasted chickpeas or edamame
- Flaxseed crackers + guacamole

PRO SNACK STRATEGIES

- **Protein first.** Even with fruit, always pair it with protein/fat.
- **Small but steady.** The goal is stabilization, not a mini-meal.
- **Plan for weak spots.** If you know 3 PM is your crash time, prep your snack ahead.
- **No naked carbs.** Crackers, fruit, or granola alone will spike you. Always pair them.

QUICK TAKEAWAY:

- **Type 1:** Snacks = safety net. Pair carbs with protein/fat.
- **Type 2:** Snacks = optional tool, not habit. Use them strategically.
- **Type 3:** Snacks = brain protectors. Prevent brain fog and mood dips.

Dinner/Supper

BEST DINNER TIMING
Type 1 Diabetes

- **When:** Consistency is key (usually **6–7:30 PM**).
- Eating too late complicates insulin dosing before bed and increases the risk of nighttime lows.
- **Pro tip:** Include protein + some slow carbs, but avoid heavy carb loads that spike late.

Type 2 Diabetes

- **When:** Earlier is better — aim for **6–7 PM**.
- Late dinners (after 8 PM) increase overnight glucose and make mornings harder (higher fasting sugar).
- **Pro tip:** If hungry later, have a small protein/fat snack instead of eating dinner at 9–10 PM.

Type 3 Diabetes (Sugar–Brain Connection)

- **When:** Earlier dinners (5:30–6:30 PM) help the brain stabilize before sleep.
- Heavy or late meals increase nighttime cortisol/adrenaline surges (panic episodes, vivid dreams).
- **Pro tip:** Prioritize protein + veggies, keep carbs light at night to avoid brain "sugar flooding" during sleep.

30 Blood Sugar–Friendly Dinner Ideas

POULTRY-BASED

1. Grilled chicken thighs + roasted Brussels sprouts + cauliflower mash
2. Turkey chili (beans optional in small portion) + avocado garnish
3. Baked chicken breast stuffed with spinach + feta, side of zucchini noodles
4. Turkey burger (no bun) + sautéed mushrooms + green beans
5. Chicken stir-fry (broccoli, cabbage, carrots, garlic) with cauliflower rice

FISH & SEAFOOD

6. Salmon fillet + asparagus + salad with olive oil
7. Shrimp stir-fry with bok choy + garlic + sesame seeds
8. Cod baked with lemon + dill + roasted broccoli
9. Tuna steak + arugula + cherry tomato salad
10. Fish tacos in lettuce wraps with avocado + salsa

BEEF & LAMB

11. Grass-fed steak + roasted mushrooms + spinach salad
12. Beef stir-fry with peppers + snow peas (served over zucchini noodles)
13. Lamb chops + grilled eggplant + Greek salad
14. Ground beef zucchini boats (stuffed with onions, peppers, cheese)
15. Slow-cooked beef stew with carrots + celery (skip potatoes or replace with turnips)

VEGETARIAN / PLANT-BASED

16. Tofu stir-fry with kale + sesame oil
17. Lentil curry with cauliflower rice
18. Chickpea & spinach stew with olive oil drizzle
19. Grilled portobello mushrooms + green beans + side salad
20. Eggplant lasagna (sliced eggplant instead of pasta)

COMFORT FOOD MADE BLOOD SUGAR FRIENDLY

21. Cauliflower-crust pizza topped with veggies + mozzarella + turkey pepperoni
22. Spaghetti squash with turkey meatballs + marinara
23. Zucchini noodles (zoodles) with pesto + grilled shrimp
24. Low-carb shepherd's pie (mashed cauliflower topping instead of potatoes)
25. Turkey lettuce wraps (ground turkey sautéed with garlic, ginger, soy sauce)

ONE-PAN / EASY MEALS

26. Sheet-pan salmon + broccoli + Brussels sprouts roasted in olive oil
27. Chicken fajita skillet (peppers, onions, avocado) — no tortillas
28. Turkey sausage + sautéed kale + roasted carrots
29. Grilled chicken or salmon over a "big salad" with avocado, olive oil, and pumpkin seeds
30. Shakshuka (eggs poached in tomato-pepper sauce) with a side of roasted zucchini

PRO TIPS FOR DINNER SUCCESS

- **Protein = anchor.** Always start with protein to stabilize blood sugar overnight.
- **Carbs at night = optional.** If you include carbs, make them slow (quinoa, beans, lentils, spaghetti squash) and small portions.
- **Don't overeat.** Large, heavy dinners spike blood sugar and stress the pancreas.
- **Type 3 especially:** Early, lighter dinners protect the brain and reduce nighttime stress episodes.

With this, you now have **30 dinners** plus timing guidelines for each diabetes type.

Desserts & Diabetes

Can You Have Any?

The Short Answer

Yes — you *can* enjoy dessert, but it has to be:

1. **Occasionally, not daily.**
2. **Paired with protein or fat.**
3. **Made from whole-food, low-glycemic ingredients.**

When dessert is reimagined this way, it doesn't have to cause massive blood sugar spikes, crashes, or cravings.

WHY TRADITIONAL DESSERTS ARE A PROBLEM

- Cake, cookies, candy = refined flour + sugar = *instant blood sugar spike.*
- Spikes = stress on the pancreas, followed by crashes (shakiness, panic, cravings).
- Over time, this worsens insulin resistance and increases the risk of Type 3 (sugar–brain connection).

THE SMARTER DESSERT STRATEGY
Rules for Dessert That Works

- **Eat it after a meal, not alone.** Your blood sugar rise will be gentler if dessert follows protein + veggies.
- **Protein/fat pairing:** Add nuts, seeds, or Greek yogurt to slow sugar release.
- **Portion awareness:** Half a cup, not half a cake.
- **Sweeten smartly:** Use low-glycemic sweeteners (stevia, monk fruit, erythritol) instead of sugar.

BLOOD SUGAR–FRIENDLY DESSERT IDEAS

FRUIT-BASED

1. Berries with whipped coconut cream (unsweetened)
2. Baked apple with cinnamon + walnuts
3. Grilled peaches with ricotta or cottage cheese
4. Chia seed pudding with unsweetened almond milk + vanilla
5. Frozen blueberries topped with warm coconut cream

CHOCOLATE FIXES

6. 85–90% dark chocolate square with almonds
7. Avocado chocolate mousse (cacao powder, avocado, stevia, vanilla)
8. Protein "hot chocolate" (unsweetened cocoa + protein powder + almond milk)
9. Greek yogurt with cacao nibs + cinnamon
10. Coconut oil fat bombs (cocoa powder + nut butter + stevia, frozen in small bites)

COOL TREATS

11. Homemade "nice cream" (frozen banana blended with almond butter & cinnamon — portion small, pair with nuts)
12. Unsweetened coconut yogurt with blueberries
13. Protein popsicles (protein powder + almond milk, frozen)
14. Strawberry smoothie bowl (with chia + almond butter, no added sugar)
15. Green tea matcha latte pops (unsweetened almond milk + matcha + stevia)

BAKED / COMFORT DESSERTS

16. Almond flour brownies (sweetened with stevia/erythritol)
17. Coconut flour muffins with walnuts
18. Pumpkin pie bites (pumpkin, almond flour crust, stevia)
19. Keto cheesecake (almond flour crust, cream cheese filling, stevia/monk fruit)
20. Zucchini chocolate chip muffins (sugar-free chocolate chips, almond flour)

BY DIABETES TYPE

- **Type 1:** Desserts are possible but must be tightly tracked with insulin dosing, always after a balanced meal.
- **Type 2:** Desserts should be low-carb and occasional. Protein/fat pairing is non-negotiable.
- **Type 3 (brain focus):** Desserts must not create sugar crashes (which worsen brain fog, panic, and memory dips). Best choices: berries, chia pudding, dark chocolate with nuts.

Key Takeaway: Dessert isn't gone — it's *different*. With the right ingredients and timing, you can still enjoy sweet moments without sabotaging your blood sugar or your brain.

The Carb Trap: Why One Slip Brings Back Cravings

What Happens During the 3-Day Reset

- In those first 72 hours without fast carbs, your body begins shifting away from running purely on quick sugar.
- Blood sugar starts to stabilize.
- Dopamine receptors in your brain begin to reset, so sugar doesn't control your reward center as strongly.
- Cravings naturally weaken.

THEN ONE SIMPLE CARB SNEAKS IN...

When you eat a cookie, a piece of white bread, or a bowl of pasta after your reset, here's what happens:

1. **Blood Sugar Spike:** Simple carbs break down fast → glucose floods your bloodstream.
2. **Insulin Surge:** Your pancreas pumps insulin to move sugar into cells.
3. **Blood Sugar Crash:** The surge overshoots → sugar levels drop too low.
4. **Brain Panic:** Your brain interprets the crash as "emergency fuel shortage" → cravings roar back.
5. **Dopamine Hit:** Sugar triggers your brain's reward pathways again, reigniting the cycle of desire → reward → crash → desire.

It's like flipping a switch that reactivates both your body's **biochemistry** and your brain's **addiction loop**.

WHY CRAVINGS FEEL SO STRONG AFTER A SLIP

- **Biological:** The crash makes your body think it needs *more* sugar immediately.
- **Neurological:** The brain remembers the "pleasure hit" and demands it again.
- **Psychological:** You may feel guilt or frustration, which increases stress (and stress drives more cravings).

THE GOOD NEWS

- **One slip doesn't erase progress.** If you get back to protein + veggies + fat right away, cravings usually fade again within 24–48 hours.
- The key is to **not let one slip turn into three days of slipping.**

HOW TO RECOVER FROM A CARB SLIP

1. **Hydrate immediately.** Water or herbal tea helps flush excess sugar.
2. **Protein + fat next meal.** Example: chicken + avocado + broccoli. This steadies blood sugar fast.
3. **Walk it out.** A 10–15 minute walk uses some of that excess glucose.
4. **Forgive yourself.** Stress raises cortisol, which *worsens* the spike-crash-craving cycle.
5. **Get back to balance.** Don't starve or "punish fast" — just resume your reset meals.

Key Takeaway: Simple carbs can pull you back into the craving cycle quickly — but you can just as quickly reset by returning to steady meals. Think of it like stepping off the path for a moment; you don't have to wander into the woods — just step back on track.

What To Do To Balance Your Blood Sugar Levels

IF YOU'VE SPIKED (BLOOD SUGAR TOO HIGH)

How it feels: Tired, foggy, thirsty, irritable, maybe a weird taste in your mouth or blurry vision.

What to do:

1. **Move your body** – a 10–20 minute brisk walk or light exercise helps muscles pull sugar out of the bloodstream.
2. **Hydrate** – drink 1–2 glasses of water; dehydration worsens high blood sugar.
3. **Protein + Veggies next meal** – skip the carbs for your next plate; focus on protein (chicken, eggs, tofu) + fiber (leafy greens).
4. **Deep breathing** – stress hormones push sugar higher. Slowing your breath calms cortisol.

IF YOU'VE CRASHED (BLOOD SUGAR TOO LOW)

How it feels: Shaky, sweaty, panicky, suddenly hungry, brain fog, racing heart.

What to do:

1. **Quick rescue if very low:** For Type 1 (or if on insulin/meds), you may need **15g fast-acting glucose** (like glucose tabs, juice, or honey). Always follow your doctor's safety plan.
2. **Stabilizer snack:** Pair a *small* carb with protein/fat to prevent rebound crash. Example: apple slices with almond butter, or half a banana with nuts.

3. **Don't overeat:** The panic makes you want to eat everything in sight — but that leads to another spike. Eat a small stabilizer, then wait 15 minutes.
4. **Track the trigger:** Skipped a meal? Too much coffee? Intense exercise? Knowing why helps prevent repeats.

EVERYDAY BALANCING HABITS (PREVENTION)

1. **Balanced Plates (50/25/25 method)** → 50% veggies, 25% protein, 25% smart carbs + healthy fat.
2. **Protein at every meal** → prevents spikes and urgent hunger.
3. **Hydrate regularly** → 6–8 cups water daily, plus herbal teas.
4. **Move after meals** → 10–15 minutes of walking is like "natural insulin."
5. **Stress resets** → breathing, prayer, meditation, or journaling calm cortisol (a hidden blood sugar driver).
6. **Steady sleep** → 7–8 hours helps hormones regulate insulin.

EMERGENCY RESET AFTER A SLIP

If you "gave in" and had cake, fries, or soda and feel the cravings roaring back:

1. **Forgive yourself.** Stress + guilt only make it worse.
2. **Drink water.** Flush out extra glucose.
3. **Protein + veggies next meal.** Reset your blood sugar within hours.
4. **Move.** A short walk right after a carb-heavy meal can cut the sugar spike in half.
5. **Wait 3 days.** If cravings hit again, remember — it takes ~3 days of steady eating to calm them.

Key Takeaway: Balancing blood sugar is about *small course corrections*, not perfection. Every spike or crash is feedback, not failure. When you respond with hydration, movement, protein, and calmness, you pull your body back into balance — and your brain will thank you.

Quick-Reference Food Lists

STABILIZERS (SUPPORT STEADY BLOOD SUGAR)

These foods release glucose slowly, reduce spikes, and support brain health.

Proteins (the anchor):

- Eggs, chicken, turkey, fish, lean beef
- Tofu, tempeh, beans, lentils
- Greek yogurt, cottage cheese

Healthy Fats (the stabilizer):

- Avocado, olives, olive oil
- Nuts & seeds (almonds, walnuts, chia, flax, pumpkin)
- Fatty fish (salmon, sardines, mackerel)
- Coconut, coconut oil (moderate amounts)

Fiber-Rich Carbs (the gentle fuel):

- Leafy greens (spinach, kale, arugula)
- Colorful veggies (broccoli, Brussels sprouts, cauliflower, peppers)
- Low-glycemic fruits (berries, apples, pears, cherries)
- Whole grains (quinoa, oats, barley, buckwheat)
- Legumes (beans, chickpeas, lentils)
- Resistant starches (cooled potatoes, green bananas, lentils)

Herbal & Spice Helpers:

- Cinnamon, turmeric, ginger, rosemary, sage

SPIKERS (CAUSE BLOOD SUGAR SURGES & CRASHES)

These foods digest quickly, flood the bloodstream with glucose, and can worsen cravings, fog, and mood swings.

Refined Carbs:

- White bread, white rice, regular pasta
- Crackers, pretzels, bagels
- Pastries, donuts, muffins

Sugary Foods & Drinks:

- Candy, chocolate bars, cookies, cake
- Soda, energy drinks, sweetened juices
- Sweetened coffee/tea drinks

High-Glycemic Fruits:

- Watermelon, pineapple, ripe bananas, grapes (in large amounts)
- Dried fruit (raisins, dates, figs — very concentrated sugar)

Other Spikers:

- Fried fast foods (fries, battered chicken, pizza)
- Processed cereals (especially "instant" or sugar-coated)
- Alcohol (especially beer, sweet cocktails, liqueurs)

If you eat a "spiker," always **pair it with a stabilizer!!!**

Conclusion: Understanding Type 3 Diabetes

Type 3 Diabetes is not yet an official diagnosis in most medical circles, but the evidence is undeniable: unstable blood sugar not only harms the body — it disrupts the brain. The same insulin resistance that clogs arteries and stresses the pancreas also starves brain cells of fuel, leading to foggy thinking, mood swings, memory lapses, and — in the long term — greater risk of dementia and Alzheimer's disease.

What makes this link so important is that it gives us a wake-up call: **the brain is not separate from blood sugar health.** Every meal, every spike, every crash sends ripples through the nervous system. For some, those ripples show up as cravings, panic, or strange "dream episodes." For others, it's word mix-ups, fatigue, or a creeping loss of mental sharpness. Over years and decades, this can add up to cognitive decline — but it doesn't have to.

The good news is that Type 3 Diabetes is not inevitable, nor is it untreatable. With every balanced meal, every mindful breath, every daily walk, and every small act of self-care, you give your brain steadier fuel and your body the chance to heal. Herbs like cinnamon, turmeric, and bitter melon can nudge the body back toward balance. Modalities like Reiki, reflexology, and meditation calm the stress response that drives blood sugar swings. And emerging science — from stem cells to artificial pancreas systems — promises a future where managing diabetes becomes easier, more precise, and more hopeful.

Type 3 Diabetes is not about labels. It's about awareness. It's about noticing the signs — the brain fog, the cravings, the sleep disturbances, the subtle memory lapses — and choosing to respond with compassion and action. It's about protecting not just your pancreas, but your mind, your clarity, and your future self.

If there is one lesson this book hopes to leave with you, it is this: **blood sugar balance is brain balance.** By caring for your glucose, you care for your energy, your memory, your mood, and your longevity. By taking steps today — however small — you can create a future where sweetness is not found in sugar, but in a sharp mind, a steady heart, and a life lived with clarity and joy.

Part VI - Recipes:

HERBAL TEAS & DRINKS FOR EACH TYPE
Type 1 Diabetes (Insulin-dependent)

(Goal: gentle support, anti-inflammatory, no extreme blood sugar swings)

1. **Fenugreek Tea**
   o Steep 1 tsp of crushed fenugreek seeds in hot water for 5–10 minutes.
   o Slows carb absorption, mild stabilizer.
2. **Ginger Tea**
   o Fresh ginger slices boiled in water for 10 min.
   o Reduces inflammation, eases digestion.
3. **Aloe Vera Drink (unsweetened, diluted)**
   o 2–3 tbsp aloe vera gel mixed in water.
   o Anti-inflammatory, may lower fasting glucose gently.
4. **Peppermint Tea**
   o Soothes digestion, supports stress relief (important for preventing cortisol-driven spikes).

Type 2 Diabetes (Insulin resistance)

(Goal: lower glucose, improve insulin sensitivity, reduce cravings)

1. **Bitter Melon Tea**
   o Sliced bitter melon steeped in boiling water for 10 min.
   o Mimics insulin's action, lowers glucose.
2. **Gymnema Tea ("Sugar Destroyer")**

- o Steep dried Gymnema leaves.
- o Reduces sugar absorption + curbs sugar cravings.
3. **Green Tea**
   - o 1–2 cups daily.
   - o Catechins improve insulin sensitivity and metabolism.
4. **Fenugreek + Cinnamon Blend**
   - o Seeds + stick simmered together.
   - o Double effect: slows absorption + improves insulin sensitivity.

Type 3 Diabetes (Sugar–Brain Connection)

(Goal: brain protection, memory support, steady glucose for cognitive clarity)

1. **Sage Tea**
   - o Fresh/dried sage leaves steeped in hot water.
   - o Improves memory, focus, and cognitive performance.
2. **Rosemary Tea**
   - o Fresh sprigs steeped 5–10 min.
   - o Boosts circulation to the brain, supports recall.
3. **Ginkgo Tea**
   - o Steep ginkgo biloba leaves (or use standardized tea bags).
   - o Enhances brain blood flow, protects neurons.
4. **Gotu Kola Tea**
   - o Mild, earthy herbal tea.
   - o Traditional "brain tonic" supports nerve/myelin health.
5. **Matcha Green Tea (powdered)**
   - o Whisked into warm water/almond milk.
   - o Antioxidants + gentle caffeine → brain clarity without crash.

PRO TIPS FOR ALL TYPES

- **Morning teas:** Green tea, matcha, or ginger (gentle energy + metabolism boost).
- **Afternoon teas:** Cinnamon, fenugreek, sage, rosemary (stabilizing + focus).
- **Evening teas:** Turmeric latte, peppermint, chamomile + cinnamon (calming + blood sugar steady overnight).

Key Takeaway:

- **Type 1:** Gentle anti-inflammatory teas (ginger, fenugreek, peppermint).
- **Type 2:** Stronger glucose regulators (bitter melon, gymnema, green tea).
- **Type 3:** Brain-protective teas (sage, rosemary, ginkgo, gotu kola).

CINNAMON TEA (CRAVING-CALMING & BLOOD SUGAR FRIENDLY)

Ingredients (1 mug):

- 1 cinnamon stick (or 1 tsp ground cinnamon)
- 1 cup hot water
- Optional: 1–2 slices of fresh ginger or a squeeze of lemon

Instructions:

1. Place the cinnamon stick (or powder) in a mug.
2. Pour boiling water over it. Let steep 10 minutes (longer = stronger flavor).
3. Add ginger slices or lemon if desired.
4. Drink warm, especially when sugar cravings hit.

Why it helps: Cinnamon improves insulin sensitivity and can give a "sweet" flavor without sugar.

WARM TURMERIC LATTE (UNSWEETENED "GOLDEN MILK")

Ingredients (1 serving):

- 1 cup unsweetened almond, coconut, or dairy milk
- ½ tsp ground turmeric
- ¼ tsp ground cinnamon
- Pinch of ground black pepper (boosts turmeric's absorption)
- Optional: pinch of ginger or cardamom

Instructions:

1. Heat milk in a small pot until warm (not boiling).
2. Whisk in turmeric, cinnamon, and black pepper until smooth.
3. Pour into a mug. Sprinkle with extra cinnamon if you like.
4. Sip slowly before bed or during an evening craving.

Why it helps: Turmeric is anti-inflammatory, cinnamon stabilizes blood sugar, and the warm ritual comforts the brain, reducing cravings.

CHAI TEA & BLOOD SUGAR
Core Ingredients & Their Effects

- **Black Tea (base):** Contains polyphenols that can **improve insulin sensitivity** and help stabilize blood sugar. Provides a gentle caffeine boost without the crash.
- **Cinnamon:** One of the best blood sugar stabilizers; improves insulin sensitivity.

- **Ginger:** Anti-inflammatory, aids digestion, lowers blood sugar modestly.
- **Cardamom:** Supports digestion and circulation; antioxidant-rich.
- **Cloves:** High in antioxidants, may improve insulin function.
- **Black Pepper:** Enhances absorption of other spices (especially turmeric if added).

How Chai Affects Each Type

- **Type 1:**
  - Can enjoy chai in moderation. The spices are beneficial, but **watch the milk and sugar.** Skip added sugar, and use unsweetened almond/coconut milk or whole milk (if tolerated).
  - Caffeine in black tea can sometimes raise blood sugar slightly, so monitor.
- **Type 2:**
  - Excellent choice if unsweetened. The spice blend is **blood sugar-friendly.**
  - Drinking chai after a carb-heavy meal may **reduce the post-meal glucose spike.**
- **Type 3 (Brain Connection):**
  - Chai supports the brain through **anti-inflammatory spices** and steady caffeine from black tea, which is gentler than coffee.
  - Cinnamon + ginger + cardamom all improve circulation and brain clarity.

The Cautions

- Most coffee shops (Starbucks, etc.) use **chai syrup** loaded with sugar → this turns a healthy tea into a sugar bomb.

- Traditional chai is often sweetened heavily with sugar or condensed milk.
- **The fix:** Make it yourself or buy sugar-free blends.

Simple Blood Sugar–Friendly Chai Recipe

1. Bring 2 cups water + ½ cup unsweetened milk (or almond/coconut milk) to a boil.
2. Add 1 cinnamon stick, 3 cardamom pods, 3 cloves, 4 slices fresh ginger, and a pinch of black pepper.
3. Simmer for 10 minutes.
4. Add 1 black tea bag (or 1 tsp loose black tea). Steep 3–5 minutes.
5. Strain and enjoy. Sweeten lightly with **stevia, monk fruit, or a dash of vanilla** if desired.

Key Takeaway:
Chai tea (when made without sugar) is a **blood sugar–balancing, brain-boosting drink** that fits all three diabetes types. It combines the power of black tea with anti-inflammatory, insulin-supporting spices.

Breakfast Recipes for Blood Sugar Balance

1. VEGGIE OMELET WITH AVOCADO

Ingredients

- 2–3 eggs (or 2 eggs + 2 egg whites)
- 1 cup spinach, peppers, mushrooms (or any veggies you have)
- ½ avocado (sliced)
- 1 tsp olive oil or butter

Instructions

1. Sauté veggies in olive oil/butter.
2. Add whisked eggs, cook until set.
3. Top with avocado slices and black pepper.

Why it works: High protein + healthy fat + fiber = no sugar spike, keeps you full for hours.

---

2. GREEK YOGURT POWER BOWL

Ingredients

- ¾ cup plain Greek yogurt (unsweetened, full fat)
- ¼ cup blueberries or raspberries
- 1 tbsp chia seeds or ground flax
- 1 tbsp walnuts or almonds
- Dash of cinnamon

Instructions

1. Stir yogurt with seeds and cinnamon.
2. Top with berries and nuts.

Why it works: Protein + fat + fiber-rich carbs = steady fuel. Cinnamon adds extra blood sugar balance.

---

3. SAVORY AVOCADO TOAST (LOW-CARB)

Ingredients

- 1 slice sprouted-grain bread *or* low-carb bread alternative
- ½ avocado, mashed
- 1 boiled or poached egg
- Sprinkle of pumpkin seeds

Instructions

1. Toast bread, spread avocado.
2. Top with egg + seeds.

Why it works: Protein + fat stabilizes the small amount of carbs. For **Types 2 or 3**, keep it to 1 slice max.

---

4. BREAKFAST SALAD WITH SMOKED SALMON

Ingredients

- 2 cups baby greens (spinach, arugula, kale)
- 2 oz smoked salmon or leftover grilled salmon
- ½ cucumber, sliced
- 1 boiled egg

- Olive oil + lemon juice dressing

Instructions

1. Toss greens, cucumber, and dressing.
2. Add salmon + egg on top.

Why it works: A lighter but protein-rich breakfast that supports both blood sugar and brain clarity.

---

5. ALMOND FLOUR PROTEIN PANCAKES

Ingredients

- ½ cup almond flour
- 2 eggs
- 2 tbsp unsweetened almond milk
- ½ tsp cinnamon
- 1 scoop vanilla protein powder (optional)
- Coconut oil for cooking

Instructions

1. Mix all ingredients into a batter.
2. Cook pancakes in coconut oil until golden.
3. Top with a few berries and a spoonful of Greek yogurt instead of syrup.

Why it works: No refined flour, high protein + fat → tastes like pancakes, but stabilizes sugar.

6. CINNAMON CHIA PUDDING (MAKE-AHEAD)

Ingredients

- 3 tbsp chia seeds
- 1 cup unsweetened almond milk
- ½ tsp cinnamon
- A few drops of stevia or monk fruit
- Topping: walnuts + blueberries

Instructions

1. Mix chia seeds, almond milk, cinnamon, and sweetener.
2. Refrigerate overnight.
3. Top with nuts + berries in the morning.

Why it works: Great prep-ahead breakfast with fiber + protein + fat to crush morning cravings.

PRO TIPS FOR BREAKFAST BALANCE

- Always anchor with **protein first** → eggs, Greek yogurt, salmon, or nuts.
- **Keep carbs smart + fibrous** → berries, veggies, quinoa, oats in moderation.
- Add **healthy fat** → avocado, olive oil, nuts, coconut, seeds.
- For **Type 3**: keep breakfast earlier + balanced to avoid mid-morning brain fog.

Lunch Recipes for Blood Sugar Balance

1. GRILLED CHICKEN & QUINOA BOWL

Ingredients

- 4 oz grilled chicken breast
- ½ cup cooked quinoa
- 1 cup roasted broccoli + zucchini
- 1 tbsp olive oil + lemon juice

Instructions

1. Layer quinoa, veggies, and chicken.
2. Drizzle olive oil + lemon dressing.

Why it works: Balanced protein, fiber/carbs, and healthy fat keep energy steady.

---

2. TURKEY & AVOCADO LETTUCE WRAPS

Ingredients

- 3–4 large romaine or butter lettuce leaves
- 4 oz sliced turkey breast
- ½ avocado, sliced
- Tomato + cucumber slices
- Mustard or hummus for spread

Instructions

1. Spread lettuce leaves, add fillings.
2. Roll up like a wrap.

Why it works: Low-carb, high protein/fat combo → no post-lunch slump.

---

3. LENTIL & VEGGIE SOUP

Ingredients

- 1 cup cooked lentils
- 2 cups vegetable broth
- 1 cup spinach + carrots + celery
- 1 tsp olive oil
- Herbs: thyme, garlic, pepper

Instructions

1. Sauté veggies in olive oil.
2. Add broth + lentils, simmer 15 min.

Why it works: Fiber-rich carbs + plant protein = slow-release energy, great for Type 2 & 3.

---

4. SALMON & SPINACH SALAD

Ingredients

- 2 cups baby spinach
- 4 oz grilled or canned salmon
- ½ avocado, diced
- 1 tbsp pumpkin seeds
- Olive oil + balsamic vinegar

Instructions

1. Toss spinach with dressing.

2. Add salmon, avocado, and seeds.

Why it works: Omega-3s protect the brain (Type 3), while protein + fat stabilize sugar.

---

5. CHICKPEA & VEGGIE POWER BOWL

Ingredients

- 1 cup roasted cauliflower + bell peppers
- ½ cup cooked chickpeas
- 2 tbsp tahini dressing
- Fresh parsley

Instructions

1. Roast veggies until golden.
2. Add chickpeas + drizzle with tahini.

Why it works: Plant protein + fiber keep blood sugar stable; tahini adds brain-boosting fats.

---

6. SHRIMP STIR-FRY (CAULIFLOWER RICE)

Ingredients

- 4 oz shrimp, peeled
- 2 cups mixed veggies (broccoli, snow peas, peppers)
- 1 cup cauliflower rice
- 1 tbsp sesame oil + garlic + ginger

Instructions

1. Stir-fry shrimp + veggies in sesame oil.

2. Serve over cauliflower rice.

Why it works: High protein, low carb, great for brain clarity after lunch.

---

7. GREEK MEZZE PLATE

Ingredients

- 4 oz grilled chicken or lamb slices
- ½ cup cucumber + tomato salad
- 2 tbsp hummus
- 4–6 olives
- Small side of roasted eggplant or zucchini

Instructions
Assemble everything on a plate mezze-style.

Why it works: Mediterranean flavors + protein + fiber + healthy fats = powerful for Type 2 & brain health.

---

8. EGG SALAD LETTUCE BOATS

Ingredients

- 2 boiled eggs, mashed with 1 tsp avocado mayo or Greek yogurt
- Lettuce leaves (romaine or butter)
- Cucumber + celery slices

Instructions
Spoon egg salad into lettuce leaves, top with crunchy veggies.

Why it works: Protein-anchored, low-carb, perfect for afternoon focus.

PRO TIPS FOR LUNCH BALANCE

- **Eat protein first.** This prevents the afternoon crash.
- **Add crunch from veggies.** They act like a natural "fiber sponge."
- **Add healthy fat.** Avocado, olive oil, nuts, tahini → signal satiety and protect brain myelin.
- **For Type 3:** Favor omega-3s (salmon, walnuts) + polyphenols (olive oil, greens) for brain clarity.

Dinner Recipes for Blood Sugar Balance

1. BAKED SALMON WITH ROASTED VEGETABLES

Ingredients

- 4–6 oz salmon fillet
- 1 cup broccoli + zucchini + carrots
- 1 tbsp olive oil
- Lemon slices + dill

Instructions

1. Place salmon and veggies on a baking sheet.
2. Drizzle with olive oil, top salmon with lemon + dill.
3. Bake at 375°F for 20 min.

Why it works: Protein + omega-3 fats protect the brain and reduce inflammation.

---

2. HERB-ROASTED CHICKEN WITH CAULIFLOWER MASH

Ingredients

- 4 oz chicken thigh or breast
- 1 cup cauliflower florets (steamed + mashed with olive oil)
- Steamed green beans

Instructions

1. Roast chicken with herbs + garlic.

2. Serve with mashed cauliflower + beans.

Why it works: Comfort food feel without the starchy potato crash.

---

3. TURKEY & VEGETABLE CHILI

Ingredients

- 6 oz ground turkey
- 1 cup kidney beans
- 1 cup chopped peppers, onions, zucchini
- Tomato base + chili spices

Instructions

1. Brown turkey, add veggies + beans.
2. Simmer with tomato + spices for 30 min.

Why it works: Protein + fiber carbs = slow release; beans feed gut microbiome.

---

4. BEEF & BROCCOLI STIR-FRY (LOW CARB)

Ingredients

- 4 oz lean beef strips
- 2 cups broccoli
- 1 tbsp coconut aminos or tamari
- 1 tsp sesame oil + garlic + ginger

Instructions

1. Stir-fry beef in sesame oil.

202 | CONSTANCE SANTEGO

2. Add broccoli + garlic + sauce, cook 5 min.

Why it works: Classic Asian dish without rice spike — use cauliflower rice if desired.

---

5. LEMON GARLIC SHRIMP WITH ZOODLES

Ingredients

- 6 oz shrimp
- 2 cups zucchini noodles (zoodles)
- Olive oil, garlic, lemon juice

Instructions

1. Sauté shrimp with garlic + oil.
2. Toss with zoodles and lemon juice.

Why it works: Low-carb pasta alternative, high in protein, light for evening digestion.

---

6. LENTIL & SPINACH CURRY (VEGETARIAN)

Ingredients

- 1 cup cooked lentils
- 2 cups spinach
- ½ cup coconut milk
- Curry spices: turmeric, cumin, coriander

Instructions

1. Simmer lentils with coconut milk + spices.
2. Add spinach at the end.

Why it works: Plant protein + fiber + anti-inflammatory spices = steady glucose + brain protection.

---

7. STUFFED BELL PEPPERS

Ingredients

- 2 bell peppers, halved
- 4 oz ground chicken or turkey
- ½ cup quinoa
- Tomato sauce + herbs

Instructions

1. Cook filling (meat + quinoa + sauce).
2. Fill peppers, bake 20 min at 375°F.

Why it works: Balanced protein + smart carbs inside a veggie "bowl."

---

8. MEDITERRANEAN BAKED COD

Ingredients

- 4 oz cod fillet
- Cherry tomatoes, olives, onions, spinach
- Olive oil + oregano

Instructions

1. Bake cod with veggies + drizzle of oil.
2. Serve warm with extra greens.

Why it works: Brain-healthy Mediterranean fats + lean protein.

Snack Ideas for Blood Sugar Balance

PROTEIN + FAT ANCHORS (BEST FOR STABILITY)

- Handful of **almonds, walnuts, or Brazil nuts**
- **Boiled egg** with cucumber slices
- **Cheese stick** + cherry tomatoes
- **Turkey or chicken roll-ups** (wrapped around avocado or cucumber)
- **Cottage cheese** with celery sticks

Why it works: Protein and fat prevent dips and crashes, calm cravings.

PROTEIN + SMART CARB COMBOS (BRAIN FUEL)

- **Apple slices + almond butter**
- **Berries + Greek yogurt (unsweetened)**
- **Half a banana + walnuts**
- **Rice cake (brown rice) + cottage cheese + cinnamon**
- **Carrot sticks + hummus**

Why it works: Pairing carbs with protein/fat prevents the sugar flood and fuels the brain steadily.

FIBER + FLAVOR BOOSTERS (CRAVING CONTROL)

- **Roasted chickpeas** with sea salt + paprika
- **Edamame** (lightly salted)
- **Flaxseed crackers + guacamole**
- **Veggie sticks** with tzatziki or hummus
- **Pumpkin seeds** roasted with cinnamon

Why it works: Fiber slows glucose absorption, while strong flavors (cinnamon, savory spices) curb cravings.

COMFORT SNACKS (WARM & CALMING)

- **Cinnamon tea** with roasted sunflower seeds
- **Warm turmeric latte** with a small handful of almonds
- **Herbal chai (unsweetened)** with a boiled egg
- **Bone broth** (protein-rich, soothing, no spike)

Why it works: Warm liquids + protein/fat reduce the brain's craving signals.

WHEN TO SNACK (BY TYPE)

- **Type 1:**
  - Snacks may be essential to prevent lows (especially overnight or before exercise).
  - Pair carbs with protein to avoid rebound spikes.
- **Type 2:**
  - Snacks are **optional** — use them strategically if meals were small, blood sugar dips, or cravings hit.
  - Avoid grazing all day; aim for **2–3 solid meals** with **1–2 stabilizing snacks** if needed.
- **Type 3 (Brain Connection):**
  - Snacks can be protective → prevent brain fog, memory lapses, or night episodes.
  - Best timing: mid-afternoon (3–4 pm) or early evening (7–8 pm) to stabilize brain fuel.

THE SNACK RULE OF THUMB: NO NAKED CARBS

What's a Naked Carb?

A *naked carb* is any carbohydrate eaten **alone** without protein, fiber, or fat. Examples:

- A banana by itself
- A handful of pretzels
- A plain slice of toast
- A glass of juice

What happens?

- Carbs break down quickly into glucose.
- With nothing to "slow them down," they hit your bloodstream fast.
- Result: **spike → crash → cravings.**

HOW TO DRESS YOUR CARBS

Pair every carb with a **protein or healthy fat** → this slows digestion, prevents blood sugar spikes, and helps your brain feel steady.

Examples:

- Apple 🍎 + almond butter 🥜
- Crackers + cheese 🧀
- Berries 🫐 + Greek yogurt 🥣
- Toast + avocado + egg 🥑🍳
- Banana 🍌 + walnuts 🌰

Now, instead of a rush of sugar, you get **steady fuel + satiety.**

WHY IT MATTERS FOR TYPE 3 DIABETES

- Naked carbs flood the brain with sugar, then leave it starving.
- This rollercoaster fuels **brain fog, vivid dreams, panic-like episodes, and memory lapses.**
- Protein + fat = a steady drip of glucose → your neurons stay fed, calm, and sharp.

QUICK SNACK FORMULAS

Think of it like a **simple equation:**

Carb (fruit, grain, starch) + Protein/Fat = Smart Snack

- Grapes + string cheese
- Carrots + hummus
- Whole-grain toast + peanut butter
- Cucumber slices + cottage cheese
- A square of dark chocolate + a handful of nuts

Key Takeaway:
Every time you reach for a snack, ask yourself:
"Am I about to eat a naked carb, or did I dress it up?"
If it's "naked," add a protein or fat — your blood sugar and your brain will thank you.

Desserts

1. CHIA SEED PUDDING

Ingredients:

- 3 tbsp chia seeds
- 1 cup unsweetened almond or coconut milk
- ½ tsp vanilla extract
- Dash of cinnamon
- Stevia or monk fruit to taste

Instructions:
Mix everything in a jar, stir well, and refrigerate overnight. Top with a few berries or nuts.

---

2. AVOCADO CHOCOLATE MOUSSE

Ingredients:

- 1 ripe avocado
- 2 tbsp unsweetened cocoa powder
- 2–3 tbsp unsweetened almond milk
- ½ tsp vanilla extract
- Stevia/monk fruit to taste

Instructions:
Blend until smooth and creamy. Chill before serving.

3. BERRIES & COCONUT CREAM

Ingredients:

- ½ cup fresh blueberries or raspberries
- 2 tbsp unsweetened coconut cream
- Dash of cinnamon

Instructions:
Whip coconut cream until fluffy, spoon over berries, and sprinkle with cinnamon.

---

4. DARK CHOCOLATE ALMOND BITES

Ingredients:

- 2 oz 85–90% dark chocolate
- ¼ cup raw almonds

Instructions:
Melt chocolate, dip almonds, and spread on parchment. Chill until hardened. Break into clusters.

---

5. CINNAMON BAKED APPLE

Ingredients:

- 1 apple, cored and sliced
- 1 tbsp chopped walnuts
- Dash of cinnamon
- Few drops of stevia (optional)

Instructions:
Bake at 350°F (175°C) for 15–20 minutes until soft. Top with walnuts.

---

6. PUMPKIN PIE CUPS

Ingredients:

- ½ cup canned pumpkin puree
- 2 tbsp almond flour
- 1 tbsp coconut oil
- ½ tsp pumpkin spice
- Stevia to taste

Instructions:
Mix, pour into a ramekin, and bake at 350°F for 20 minutes. Tastes like mini pumpkin pie.

---

7. GREEK YOGURT PARFAIT

Ingredients:

- ½ cup plain Greek yogurt (full fat)
- 1 tbsp chia seeds
- 2 tbsp walnuts or pecans
- ¼ cup berries
- Dash of cinnamon

Instructions:
Layer in a glass for a parfait effect.

8. KETO CHEESECAKE CUPS

Ingredients:

- 4 oz cream cheese (softened)
- 2 tbsp sour cream
- 1 tbsp almond flour
- ½ tsp vanilla extract
- Stevia/monk fruit to taste

Instructions:
Mix, spoon into muffin cups, bake at 325°F (160°C) for 12–15 min. Chill before eating.

---

9. COCONUT FAT BOMBS

Ingredients:

- ¼ cup coconut oil (melted)
- 2 tbsp almond butter
- 1 tbsp cocoa powder
- Stevia/monk fruit to taste

Instructions:
Mix, pour into silicone molds or ice cube tray, freeze until solid.

10. ZUCCHINI CHOCOLATE MUFFINS

Ingredients:

- 1 cup grated zucchini (squeezed dry)
- 1 cup almond flour
- 2 tbsp cocoa powder
- 2 eggs
- 2 tbsp coconut oil
- ½ tsp baking powder
- Stevia/monk fruit to taste

Instructions:
Mix, spoon into muffin tin, bake at 350°F (175°C) for 20–25 minutes.

PRO TIPS FOR DESSERT SUCCESS

- Always pair with **protein or fat** (yogurt, nuts, coconut cream) to blunt blood sugar rise.
- Keep portions small — ½ cup or 1 piece is plenty.
- Enjoy **after a meal, not as a stand-alone snack**.

7-Day Balance Plan: Food, Movement & Mindfulness

A sample week to stabilize blood sugar, calm the brain, and restore energy. Adjust portions, timing, and intensity for your needs — this is a guide, not a prescription.

DAY 1 – GENTLE RESET

- **Breakfast:** Greek yogurt with chia seeds, blueberries, and a sprinkle of cinnamon.
- **Lunch:** Grilled chicken salad with leafy greens, avocado, olive oil, and lemon.
- **Dinner:** Salmon, roasted Brussels sprouts, and quinoa.
- **Snack:** Apple slices + almond butter.
- **Movement:** 10-minute walk after lunch and dinner.
- **Mindfulness:** 5 deep breaths before each meal → notice colors, smells, and gratitude.

DAY 2 – ENERGY & CALM

- **Breakfast:** Veggie omelet (spinach, peppers, onions) + half an avocado.
- **Lunch:** Lentil soup + side salad with olive oil.
- **Dinner:** Turkey stir-fry with broccoli, cauliflower rice, and sesame oil.
- **Snack:** Carrot sticks + hummus.
- **Movement:** Light strength training (bodyweight squats, wall push-ups, stretching).
- **Mindfulness:** Evening chamomile tea + write three things you're grateful for.

DAY 3 – SWEET BALANCE

- **Breakfast:** Overnight oats (steel-cut oats, chia, almond milk, walnuts, cinnamon).
- **Lunch:** Tuna salad with arugula, cucumber, tomatoes, olive oil dressing.
- **Dinner:** Baked chicken thighs, roasted asparagus, and sweet potato (cooled/reheated).
- **Snack:** Berries + cottage cheese.
- **Movement:** 20-minute brisk walk or dance session.
- **Mindfulness:** 5-minute meditation: *"I release fear. I welcome balance."*

DAY 4 – BRAIN NOURISHMENT

- **Breakfast:** Green smoothie (spinach, cucumber, avocado, unsweetened protein powder).
- **Lunch:** Quinoa bowl with black beans, roasted zucchini, salsa, and lime.
- **Dinner:** Grilled shrimp with sautéed kale and garlic, side of roasted cauliflower.
- **Snack:** Handful of walnuts + 1 square dark chocolate (85%).
- **Movement:** Gentle yoga or tai chi (20 minutes).
- **Mindfulness:** Journaling prompt → *"Where do I find sweetness beyond sugar?"*

DAY 5 – STRENGTH & STABILITY

- **Breakfast:** Scrambled eggs with mushrooms + side of sautéed spinach.
- **Lunch:** Turkey lettuce wraps with avocado, peppers, and tahini dressing.
- **Dinner:** Beef and vegetable stew with carrots, celery, and green beans.
- **Snack:** Celery sticks with peanut butter.

- **Movement:** 15-minute strength training (resistance bands or light weights).
- **Mindfulness:** Evening Reiki hand placement over pancreas + brain → visualize golden light.

DAY 6 – GENTLE DETOX

- **Breakfast:** Chia pudding with coconut milk, cinnamon, and sliced almonds.
- **Lunch:** Grilled salmon with arugula, roasted beet, and goat cheese salad.
- **Dinner:** Chicken curry with cauliflower rice and sautéed green beans.
- **Snack:** Green banana (small, slightly unripe) with sunflower seeds.
- **Movement:** Nature walk (30 minutes, moderate pace).
- **Mindfulness:** Gratitude walk → notice three things in nature that bring you peace.

DAY 7 – REST & RENEWAL

- **Breakfast:** Vegetable frittata with zucchini, tomato, and herbs.
- **Lunch:** Lentil + vegetable stew, side of mixed greens.
- **Dinner:** Baked cod with garlic butter, roasted carrots, and quinoa.
- **Snack:** Cottage cheese with cinnamon and a few blueberries.
- **Movement:** Gentle stretching or restorative yoga (15–20 minutes).
- **Mindfulness:** Reflection journaling → *"How did my energy feel this week? What foods, movements, or practices made me feel most balanced?"*

Part VII - Natural/Alternative Medicine

Ayurveda, TCM & Other Traditional Approaches for Diabetes

AYURVEDA (INDIA'S TRADITIONAL MEDICINE)

In Ayurveda, diabetes is often described as **"Madhumeha"** (honey urine disease). The root imbalance is usually in **Kapha dosha** (too much heaviness, sluggish digestion, excess sweetness), but Pitta and Vata can also be involved.

Ayurvedic Strategies:

- **Herbs**
  - Gymnema sylvestre (Gurmar = "sugar destroyer")** – reduces sugar absorption in the gut, decreases cravings.
  - **Fenugreek seeds** – fiber-rich, stabilize blood sugar.
  - **Bitter gourd (Karela / Bitter melon)** – insulin-mimicking effect.
  - **Neem leaves** – bitter tonic, supports the pancreas.
  - **Turmeric** – reduces inflammation, supports the liver and pancreas.
- **Lifestyle**

- o Wake early, daily movement (yoga + walking).
- o Gentle fasting or spacing meals to rest digestion.
- o Avoid day-sleeping (linked with Kapha imbalance).
- **Diet**
  - o Emphasize bitter, astringent, and pungent foods (greens, legumes, spices).
  - o Reduce sweet, heavy, oily foods (bread, rice, sugar, fried foods).
- **Yoga & Breathwork**
  - o **Kapalabhati pranayama** (breath of fire) stimulates the pancreas.
  - o Gentle yoga postures that massage the abdomen (twists, forward bends).

TRADITIONAL CHINESE MEDICINE (TCM)

In TCM, diabetes is called **"Xiao Ke"** (wasting & thirsting disorder). It is usually seen as an imbalance in the **Spleen & Stomach (digestion)**, with involvement of **Kidney Yin deficiency** over time (leading to fatigue, dryness, aging).

TCM Strategies:

- **Herbs**
  - o **Bitter melon (Ku Gua)** – clears "heat," lowers sugar.
  - o **Ginseng (Ren Shen)** – boosts Qi, supports energy, and the pancreas.
  - o **Licorice root (Gan Cao)** – harmonizes other herbs, supports adrenal balance.
  - o **Rehmannia (Shu Di Huang)** – nourishes Yin, supports the kidneys (common in long-term diabetes).
  - o **Astragalus (Huang Qi)** – improves energy, immune function, and reduces fatigue.
- **Acupuncture**

> o Points like **ST36 (Zusanli)** and **SP6 (Sanyinjiao)** support digestion, energy, and blood sugar regulation.

- **Lifestyle**
  - o Balance meals with warm, cooked foods.
  - o Avoid excess cold/raw foods (hard on digestion).
  - o Stress reduction — meditation, Qi Gong, Tai Chi to calm cortisol.

OTHER TRADITIONAL APPROACHES
Unani Medicine (Persian/Arabic Tradition)

- Diabetes is seen as excess "heat" and "sweetness" in the blood.
- Herbs: fenugreek, black cumin seed, Indian kino tree (Pterocarpus marsupium).

Indigenous/Herbal Traditions

- **North America:** Blueberry leaf tea, cedar tea, prickly pear cactus (nopal) for blood sugar balance.
- **Africa:** Moringa leaf, baobab fruit powder (fiber-rich, antioxidant).

MODERN RESEARCH OVERLAP

What's fascinating is that many of these traditional remedies (gymnema, fenugreek, bitter melon, turmeric, ginseng) are now **clinically studied** and show real measurable effects on:

- Lowering fasting glucose
- Improving insulin sensitivity
- Reducing A1c
- Supporting brain function

Key Takeaway:

- **Ayurveda** emphasizes bitter herbs, yoga, and Kapha-balancing diets.
- **TCM** focuses on supporting digestion (Spleen/Stomach) and kidney Yin with herbs, acupuncture, and Qi Gong.
- **Other traditions** add local plants like prickly pear, moringa, or blueberry leaves.
- None replace medication if required, but all can **support stability, reduce complications, and improve quality of life.**

Holistic Modalities for Blood Sugar Balance & Brain Health

REIKI (ENERGY HEALING)

- **How it helps:**
  - Calms the nervous system, reducing cortisol and adrenaline spikes (both raise blood sugar).
  - Restores balance in the body's energy centers (especially solar plexus chakra — linked to pancreas and digestion).
  - Promotes deep relaxation → better sleep, steadier glucose overnight.
- **Best for:** Stress-driven spikes, Type 3 (brain fog, mood swings).
- **Practical use:** Daily self-Reiki on solar plexus, or sessions focused on pancreas + adrenal balance.

REFLEXOLOGY (FOOT/HAND THERAPY)

- **How it helps:**
  - o Specific points on the feet correspond to the **pancreas, liver, kidneys, and brain.**
  - o Stimulating these zones improves circulation, balances hormones, and supports organ function.
  - o Calms the nervous system → steadier blood sugar.
- **Best for:** All types, especially Type 2 (organ stress) and Type 3 (brain support).
- **Practical use:** Pressing the pancreas reflex (inner arch of left foot) and solar plexus reflex (center of foot) daily.

AROMATHERAPY (ESSENTIAL OILS)

- **How it helps:**
  - o Certain oils reduce cravings, balance mood, and calm stress hormones.
  - o **Cinnamon bark & clove** → improve insulin sensitivity.
  - o **Grapefruit & peppermint** → reduce sugar cravings.
  - o **Lavender & frankincense** → reduce stress and inflammation, protect brain.
- **Best for:** Curbing cravings, stress relief, mental clarity.
- **Practical use:** Inhalation during cravings, diffuser blends, diluted oils massaged on abdomen/soles of feet.

MEDITATION, BREATHWORK & VISUALIZATION

- **How it helps:**
  - o Meditation lowers cortisol → less sugar dumped into bloodstream.
  - o Breathwork (like alternate nostril breathing or box breathing) balances the nervous system.
  - o Visualization: imagining the pancreas glowing and balanced → creates a mind-body healing response.
- **Best for:** Stress spikes, Type 3 (episodes with vivid dreams or memory fog).

MASSAGE THERAPY

- **How it helps:**
  - o Improves circulation → prevents complications like neuropathy.
  - o Reduces muscle tension and stress hormones.
  - o Enhances insulin absorption for those injecting insulin in fatty tissue.
- **Best for:** Type 1 (circulation), Type 2 (stress/weight), Type 3 (relaxation, brain clarity).

ACUPRESSURE & ACUPUNCTURE

- **How it helps:**
  - o Stimulates meridians linked to the pancreas, stomach, spleen, and kidney.
  - o Reduces cravings and stabilizes digestion.
  - o Improves insulin sensitivity in Type 2.
- **Best for:** All types, especially Type 2 & 3.
- **Example points:** SP6 (Sanyinjiao), ST36 (Zusanli), LI11 (Quchi).

OTHER MODALITIES

- **Yoga:** Twists and forward bends massage the pancreas, and pranayama reduces stress.
- **Sound Therapy:** Tuning forks (weighted over solar plexus, pancreas reflex points) can calm the nervous system and regulate energy flow.
- **Hydrotherapy:** Warm foot baths improve circulation in diabetics with neuropathy.

Key Takeaway

- **Reiki**: balances energy, calms stress hormones.
- **Reflexology**: stimulates pancreas + brain zones.
- **Aromatherapy**: curbs cravings, reduces stress.
- **Meditation/Breathwork**: lowers cortisol + supports the brain.
- **Massage/Acupressure/Yoga**: improve circulation, digestion, and insulin sensitivity.

When combined with nutrition, hydration, and movement, these modalities **create a full-body healing approach** that supports not just blood sugar but **emotional + spiritual balance**.

Nighttime Rituals & Dream Science

WHY NIGHT MATTERS SO MUCH

Night is when the body and brain repair, restore, and reset. Blood sugar fluctuations don't stop when you sleep — in fact, they may show up most clearly at night: in **vivid dreams, sudden wake-ups, racing heart, or 3 AM "liver dumps."**

Sleep is also when the brain clears toxins through the **glymphatic system,** processes memories, and strengthens learning. If blood sugar is unstable, this cleansing and organizing process is interrupted — leading to brain fog, forgetfulness, and fatigue.

THE SCIENCE OF DREAMS & BLOOD SUGAR

Sleep is not just "off time" — it's a highly active state where your brain is repairing, reorganizing, and communicating with the body. Blood sugar balance plays a huge role in how well this process works.

HIGH SUGAR BEFORE BED

When you go to bed with elevated blood sugar:

- Your body works overtime to process the excess glucose.
- This keeps your nervous system more "alert," making it harder to drift into deep sleep.
- You may experience **restless tossing, vivid or fragmented dreams, and frequent bathroom trips** (as the kidneys try to flush out sugar).
- Dreams during these nights often feel **busy, chaotic, or disconnected,** reflecting the brain's struggle to organize under stress.

LOW SUGAR DURING SLEEP

If your sugar dips too low overnight (especially if you skipped dinner, exercised late, or had too much medication):

- Your body releases **adrenaline and cortisol** to rescue you.
- This "fight-or-flight" surge can trigger **panic-like dreams, night sweats, trembling, or sudden waking.**
- Dreams may feel intense, scary, or urgent — because your brain is literally crying out for fuel.
- These episodes can leave you drained, anxious, and exhausted the next morning.

BALANCED BLOOD SUGAR = BALANCED DREAMS

When your glucose is steady before bed:

- Your brain cycles naturally through **deep sleep and REM sleep** (the dream-rich stage).
- **REM sleep** is when memories are consolidated, emotions are processed, and creativity flourishes.
- Dreams during balanced nights often feel more **coherent, symbolic, or insightful** because the brain has the fuel it needs to process calmly.
- This balance supports **better memory, sharper focus, and more emotional resilience** the next day.

WHY DREAMS MATTER FOR HEALING

Dreams are not random. They are the brain's way of:

- **Sorting** the day's experiences.
- **Healing** emotional stress by replaying or reframing events.
- **Communicating** body needs — sometimes showing up as strange or symbolic messages when sugar levels swing.

When you pay attention to your dreams, you gain insight not just into your mind, but into your body's sugar rhythms.

Your dreams are part of your health story. Chaotic, panic-filled nights may reflect unstable blood sugar, while calmer, symbolic dreams often signal balance. Tracking both your **dream patterns** and your **food/stress habits** gives you powerful clues about how your body and brain are working together.

NIGHTTIME RITUALS FOR STEADY SLEEP

1. The Last Meal Matters

- Finish eating **2–3 hours before bed.**
- Choose **protein + healthy fat + non-starchy veggies.**
- If you tend to crash at night: add a **light protein snack** (boiled egg, cottage cheese with cinnamon, or nut butter on celery).

2. Calming Teas & Tonics

- **Chamomile or lavender tea** → relaxes nerves.
- **Cinnamon tea** → stabilizes blood sugar.
- **Golden milk (turmeric + ginger)** → anti-inflammatory, calming.

3. Prepare the Mind

- **Breathing ritual:** Inhale 4, hold 2, exhale 6 (repeat 5 times).
- **Journaling:** Release worries onto paper before bed.
- **Prayer or gratitude:** Shift the mind from stress to peace.

4. Energy Practices

- **Reiki hand placement:** Over the heart or pancreas for 5 minutes.
- **Visualization:** Imagine your blood sugar waves flattening into a calm lake.
- **Affirmation:** *"I release today. I welcome rest. My body restores itself as I sleep."*

5. Sleep Environment

- Cool, dark room.
- No screens 1 hour before bed (blue light delays melatonin).
- Keep water by the bed — thirst may be an early sugar signal.

DREAM SCIENCE & HEALING PRACTICE

Your dreams are not random — they are **feedback loops** between body and brain.

- **Keep a dream journal:** Write down dreams immediately upon waking. Look for patterns connected to meals, stress, or nighttime sugar swings.
- **Notice symbols:** Fear dreams may point to low sugar. Busy, racing dreams may link to high sugar.
- **Ask before sleep:** "What is my body trying to tell me tonight?" Let your subconscious speak.

Why This Matters
Night is not just rest — it is medicine. Stable blood sugar + soothing rituals = deeper sleep, clearer dreams, and sharper memory. Over time, nighttime peace becomes daytime clarity.

Meditation for Type 3 Healing: Calming the Sugar–Brain Connection

Why This Matters
This meditation helps calm the stress hormones that trigger sugar spikes, sends healing intention to the pancreas and brain, and reminds you that sweetness can be found beyond sugar — in balance, clarity, and peace.

(Find a quiet place. Sit comfortably, feet on the floor or cross-legged. Rest your hands in your lap. Take a slow, deep breath in, and begin...)

While your eyes remain open, allow your gaze to soften. Let the words on the page come into focus, then blur slightly, as if you are looking *through* the text instead of directly at it. You don't need to read with sharp concentration — simply let your eyes relax, letting the rhythm of the words guide you. As you continue, imagine each sentence not only as something you read, but as something you *experience* in your body. Let your mind wander into the images, your breath slow with the flow of the words, and your whole being gently settle into a state of calm awareness.

Imagine a soft golden light above your head — maybe the color of sunlight just before sunset, but know any will do.
As you breathe in, let that light gently pour down over your forehead, shoulders, chest, and belly.
With each exhale, feel your body relax a little more deeply into your chair, into this moment.

Place one hand over your heart, and one hand over your belly. Take a slow breath in for a count of **4** … hold gently for **2** … then exhale for **6.**

With each breath, imagine your blood sugar levels smoothing out like gentle waves on a calm lake.

Continue this rhythm two more times.

Now, bring your awareness to the area just below your ribs, on your left side — your pancreas.
See it bathed in soft, golden light. Whisper silently:
"You are safe. You are supported. You can rest and rejuvenate."

Now move your awareness upward, to your head. Picture your brain glowing softly, every nerve wrapped in a healthy, protective sheath of light. Whisper silently:
"You are nourished. You are steady. You are clear. Neurons move freely."

Think of any worries you've carried about your blood sugar, your memory, or your health.
With your next exhale, imagine those worries leaving your body as dark smoke.
As you inhale, see them replaced by bright, healing light.
Say silently:
"I release fear. I welcome balance."

Visualize yourself surrounded by a gentle field of light, holding your body in safety.
Picture yourself living with steady energy, sharp memory, and a peaceful heart.
Repeat silently:
"Sweetness flows through me — not from sugar, but from life itself."
Two more times...

Take one more deep breath in ... and slowly out.
When you feel ready, open your eyes. Notice how your body

feels a little steadier, your mind a little clearer, your spirit a little lighter.

The Sweetness of Life

Sometimes what we think of as a sugar craving is really a **soul craving;** our bodies call out for "sweetness," but what they may truly be asking for is comfort, joy, connection, or rest.

Food is the quickest way the brain knows to deliver that sensation — a rush of glucose lights up the reward centers, giving temporary relief. But as Louise Hay reminds us, diabetes is not about sugar alone; it reflects a deeper longing: the absence of joy, the sweetness of life withheld or forgotten.

True sweetness is not found in candy, soda, or bread. It's found in a hug, a walk in the sun, laughter with a friend, a quiet prayer, or a moment of beauty. When you pause and ask yourself, *"What am I really hungry for?"* you may find that the craving is not for sugar at all — but for kindness, love, peace, or joy.

By giving yourself sweetness in these deeper ways — the sweetness of presence, connection, gratitude, and love — the pull of sugar begins to loosen, and balance becomes more natural. In this way, healing becomes not just about food, but about filling your life with joy.

AFFIRMATIONS FOR WELCOMING THE SWEETNESS OF LIFE

Read these aloud, or silently in your heart. Let each one sink in, like a gentle medicine for both body and soul.

- I allow the sweetness of life to flow through me now.
- I nourish myself with joy, peace, and love.

- I am safe to let go of the past and open to the beauty of today.
- Every breath I take fills me with calm, clarity, and energy.
- My body digests life with ease, balance, and harmony.
- I replace sugar with the sweetness of spirit, connection, and gratitude.
- I am gentle with myself as I heal, one choice at a time.
- My brain is clear, my heart is light, and my life is full of joy.
- I welcome love, laughter, and new beginnings into every cell of my body.
- I choose balance. I choose life. I choose sweetness.

AFFIRMATION MEDITATION: WELCOMING THE SWEETNESS OF LIFE

(Find your comfortable place. Feet grounded, hands resting softly in your lap. Let your eyes relax as you read these words — not sharp or focused, but soft, as if you are seeing through the page. Allow each affirmation to land like a gentle ripple in your body, mind, and spirit.)

Take a slow, deep breath in ... and let it out.
Again — in ... and out.

As you breathe, let these words move through you:

- *I allow the sweetness of life to flow through me now.*
- *I nourish myself with joy, peace, and love.*

Breathe in gently ... breathe out slowly.

Place one hand on your heart. Feel it beating, steady, alive.
Whisper silently:

- *I am safe to let go of the past and open to the beauty of today.*

Now rest your hand on your belly. With each rise and fall of your breath, say:

- *Every breath I take fills me with calm, clarity, and energy.*

Imagine a soft glow surrounding your whole body — a gentle, protective light. In this light, let these affirmations flow through your mind like a mantra:

- *I replace sugar with the sweetness of spirit, connection, and gratitude.*
- *My brain is clear, my heart is light, and my life is full of joy.*
- *I welcome love, laughter, and new beginnings into every cell of my body.*

Stay with this for a few breaths. Imagine that with each inhale, you are filling your cells with sweetness — not from food, but from life itself. With each exhale, you are releasing fear, stress, and cravings.

To close, repeat softly, three times in your heart:

- *I choose balance. I choose life. I choose sweetness.*

Take one last deep breath in ... and gently release it.
When you are ready, lift your gaze back to the present moment — calm, steady, renewed.

REFLECTION PROMPTS

- Where do you find sweetness beyond sugar — in relationships, nature, creativity, or spirit?
- What would you tell your younger self about balance, cravings, and joy?
- What memory or hope makes you want to protect your brain and health for the future?

Journaling Questions for Reflection & Awareness

PART I –OUR WAKE-UP CALL

- What was your very first memory of feeling shaky, foggy, or "not myself" after eating?
- When has your body tried to warn you through dreams, exhaustion, or cravings — and did you listen?
- How have your loved ones noticed your symptoms before you did?

PART II – UNDERSTANDING BLOOD SUGAR & THE BRAIN

- What are three ways your brain signals you when your blood sugar is too high or too low?
- Which symptoms from the checklist (shakiness, brain fog, vision changes, strange tastes, etc.) do you experience most often?
- How do you feel when you think of the link between diabetes and Alzheimer's — fearful, motivated, hopeful?

PART III – NATURAL BLOOD SUGAR BALANCE

- What foods make you feel steady, clear, and calm?
- Which foods cause you to crash, crave, or feel foggy?
- How do you usually respond to sugar cravings — do you feed them, fight them, or pause to reflect?
- What small changes could you make this week using the 50/25/25 method?
- How does your mood change after walking, stretching, or gentle exercise?

PART IV – LIVING WITH DIABETES IN THE REAL WORLD

- How do stress and emotions (anger, grief, fear, excitement) affect your eating habits or cravings?
- What bedtime routine helps you sleep more peacefully and avoid nighttime episodes?
- How do you usually handle holidays, travel, or eating out — and what could you do differently?

HEALING & EMPOWERMENT

- If "sweetness of life" isn't about sugar, where do you find it? (Connection, joy, creativity, nature, prayer?)
- What gives you hope about your brain health and future?
- What is one empowering belief you can replace for every fearful thought you hold about diabetes?

Appendix

Lifestyle Tools for Type 2 & Type 3 Diabetes

These are not quick fixes — they are steady practices that, over time, retrain your body and brain toward balance. Think of them as the tools you keep in your health "toolbox," ready to use daily.

1. FOOD AS MEDICINE

- **Balanced plates** (50/25/25 method).
- **Food order** (veggies → protein/fat → carbs).
- **Fiber first** (slows spikes).
- **Smart swaps** (sparkling water instead of soda, berries instead of sweets).
- **Herbal & nutrient supports** (cinnamon, turmeric, bitter melon, magnesium).

2. MOVEMENT AS MEDICINE

- **Walk after meals** (lowers glucose like a gentle medication).
- **Strength training** (muscle acts as a glucose sponge).
- **Gentle exercise** (yoga, stretching, tai chi for stress + insulin sensitivity).
- **Consistency over intensity** (15 minutes daily > 1 hour once a week).

3. STRESS MANAGEMENT

- **Breathwork** (box breathing, 4-7-8).
- **Meditation / Reiki** to calm cortisol.
- **Journaling prompts** to process emotions instead of storing them.
- **Prayer or gratitude** to shift focus from fear to peace.

4. SLEEP & RHYTHM

- **Consistent bedtime** (signals hormones to reset).
- **Light protein snack before bed** (prevents crashes).
- **Bedtime rituals** (chamomile tea, lavender, meditation).
- **Limit screens before bed** (blue light blocks melatonin).

5. HYDRATION & KIDNEYS

- **Water goal:** Pale yellow urine = hydrated.
- **Kidney-support teas:** nettle, dandelion root, cinnamon.
- **Spacing fluids** (not chugging at once).

6. BRAIN & MEMORY SUPPORTS

- **Mental movement:** reading, puzzles, learning new skills.
- **Herbs:** rosemary, sage, and ginkgo for memory support.
- **Connection:** conversations, laughter, community (protects against dementia).

7. TRACKING & AWARENESS

- **Blood sugar meter or CGM** (learn patterns, not just numbers).
- **Lab markers** (fasting insulin, HOMA-IR, C-peptide, hs-CRP, B12).
- **Food & mood journal** (see how meals, sleep, and stress affect you).

Emergency Toolkit: Highs, Lows, Stress & Travel

Diabetes doesn't just live in the lab or doctor's office — it shows up in real life, sometimes when you least expect it. Having a simple **toolkit** gives you confidence and calm in the moment.

WHEN BLOOD SUGAR DROPS (HYPOGLYCEMIA / LOWS)

Symptoms: shakiness, sweating, sudden hunger, panic, dizziness, confusion.

What to Do:

1. **Check your sugar** (if possible).
2. **Follow the 15–15 Rule:** Take 15 g fast-acting carb (e.g., glucose tabs, ½ cup juice, 1 tbsp honey), wait 15 minutes, re-check.
3. Always **pair with protein/fat** afterward (e.g., nut butter, cheese, boiled egg) to prevent another crash.
4. **Emergency:** If severe (confused, faint, or unable to swallow) → call 911.

Toolkit Items: glucose tablets or gel, small juice box, protein bar, nut butter packets.

WHEN BLOOD SUGAR SPIKES (HYPERGLYCEMIA / HIGHS)

Symptoms: thirst, frequent urination, dry mouth, blurry vision, fatigue, irritability.

What to Do:

1. **Check your sugar.**
2. **Hydrate** (water, herbal tea). This helps flush excess glucose through the kidneys.
3. **Move gently.** A short walk can lower sugar without stressing the body.
4. **Check meds.** If you're prescribed insulin or oral meds, follow your doctor's correction plan.
5. **Emergency:** If sugar stays >300 mg/dL (16.7 mmol/L) with nausea/vomiting or fruity breath → ER (possible ketoacidosis).

Toolkit Items: water bottle, herbal teas (cinnamon, dandelion), walking shoes.

WHEN STRESS HITS (EMOTIONAL OR PHYSICAL)

Why: Stress hormones (cortisol, adrenaline) trigger the liver to dump glucose into the blood.

What to Do:

1. Pause. **3 slow breaths** (in for 4, hold 2, out for 6).
2. Move your body — a 5–10 min walk, stretch, or even shaking out arms/legs.
3. **Re-center:** Journal, pray, or use a calming affirmation (*"I am safe. I release fear. I welcome balance."*)
4. Hydrate. Dehydration + stress = higher sugar.

Toolkit Items: calming tea bags (chamomile, holy basil), journal + pen, breath/meditation app on phone.

WHEN TRAVELING

Travel = different time zones, food choices, and stress. Plan ahead:

Food:

- Pack stabilizers: nuts, seeds, protein bars, jerky, and herbal teas.
- Avoid "naked carbs" (fruit or crackers alone). Always pair with protein/fat.

Movement:

- Walk the airport, stretch on the plane, or do light bodyweight exercises in the hotel.
- Keep circulation moving to prevent spikes + protect heart health.

Stress & Sleep:

- Jet lag = blood sugar rollercoaster. Adjust meal timing slowly.
- Pack an eye mask, earplugs, and calming tea for better rest.

Toolkit Items: portable snacks, refillable water bottle, small walking shoes, supplements/meds in carry-on (never checked luggage).

Why This Matters
Life will always throw curves: a missed meal, an unexpected stress, a holiday, a red-eye flight. With a simple toolkit in place,

you don't have to panic. You can respond calmly, protect your brain and body, and get back into balance.

The Smart Lab Guide: Beyond Blood Sugar

When it comes to diabetes, most people are only told about two numbers: **fasting glucose** and **HbA1c.** These are important, but they don't give the full picture. Many people can have "normal" blood sugar yet already be developing **insulin resistance, inflammation, or nerve damage** that won't show up until years later.

That's why a smarter approach looks at a **full panel of markers** — not just sugar, but how your body is *using* sugar, how much stress your cells are under, and how your brain and nerves are being affected.

1. FASTING INSULIN

- **What it measures:** How much insulin your pancreas pumps out when you haven't eaten.
- **Why it matters:** High fasting insulin is one of the **earliest signs of insulin resistance** — often years before fasting glucose rises.
- **Goal:** Lower end of normal (around 2–8 µIU/mL, depending on lab).

2. HOMA-IR (INSULIN RESISTANCE SCORE)

- **What it measures:** A calculation using fasting insulin + fasting glucose.
- **Why it matters:** Shows how resistant your cells are to insulin.
- **Goal:** <2 is considered healthy; higher numbers suggest resistance.

3. C-PEPTIDE

- **What it measures:** How much insulin your pancreas is producing.
- **Why it matters:**
  - Low = pancreas not making enough insulin (common in Type 1 or "burned-out" Type 2).
  - High = pancreas is overworking to keep up with resistance.
- **Goal:** Balanced in the mid-range.

4. HS-CRP (HIGH-SENSITIVITY C-REACTIVE PROTEIN)

- **What it measures:** Inflammation in the body.
- **Why it matters:** Chronic inflammation is linked to **insulin resistance, cardiovascular risk, and brain decline.**
- **Goal:** <1 mg/L = low inflammation.

5. HOMOCYSTEINE & VITAMIN B12

- **What it measures:**
  - **Homocysteine** = amino acid linked to vascular and brain health.
  - **B12** = vital for myelin sheath (nerve insulation) and energy.
- **Why it matters:**

- o   High homocysteine = higher risk of dementia, nerve damage.
- o   Low B12 = fatigue, memory problems, neuropathy (common if on metformin).
- **Goal:** Homocysteine <10 μmol/L, B12 in healthy upper range.

6. CONTINUOUS GLUCOSE MONITORING (CGM)

- **What it is:** A small sensor worn on the skin, measuring glucose in real time (Dexcom, Libre, Eversense).
- **Why it matters:** Shows **patterns** instead of snapshots. You'll see:
  - o   How specific meals affect you.
  - o   Whether you spike after "healthy" foods.
  - o   Nighttime lows or highs you never knew about.
- **Goal:** Spend most of the day in **"time in range" (70–140 mg/dL)** with minimal spikes.

7. OTHER HELPFUL LABS

- **Triglyceride-to-HDL ratio:** Simple blood test ratio; high ratio = insulin resistance risk.
- **Liver enzymes (ALT, AST):** High levels can signal fatty liver (often paired with diabetes).
- **Kidney function (microalbumin/creatinine):** Early marker for diabetic nephropathy.

SMART LAB TAKEAWAY

Don't settle for "Your sugar looks fine." Ask for the deeper labs. Each one tells a part of the story:

- **Fasting insulin & HOMA-IR** → how resistant are you?
- **C-peptide** → is your pancreas coping or failing?
- **hs-CRP** → is inflammation making it worse?

- **Homocysteine & B12** → are your nerves and brain at risk?
- **CGM** → what's *really* happening day to day?

Key Takeaway: These labs don't just measure your sugar — they measure your *future.* By looking deeper, you can take action earlier, protect your pancreas, and safeguard your brain against Type 3 Diabetes.

What an Apple Watch *Cannot* Do on Its Own

Despite rumors, **no Apple Watch or smartwatch is currently capable of directly measuring blood glucose** through the skin. The FDA has explicitly cautioned against using any smartwatch or ring claiming to monitor blood sugar levels without piercing the skin—these are not approved and may be dangerously inaccurate.

HOW THE APPLE WATCH *CAN* DISPLAY BLOOD SUGAR: USING CGM SYSTEMS
Continuous Glucose Monitors (CGMs)

The Apple Watch *can* show your glucose readings—**but only** when paired with an **FDA-approved Continuous Glucose Monitor (CGM)** like the **Dexcom G6 or G7** or **Abbott's FreeStyle Libre**. These CGMs use a tiny sensor inserted under the skin to measure interstitial glucose levels.

- The **Dexcom G7**, for instance, can now connect *directly* to your Apple Watch without needing an iPhone nearby, offering real-time glucose data via Bluetooth.
- There are convenient Apple Watch apps like **GlucoWatch** (for Libre devices) and **Gluroo** (for Dexcom/Libre) that display glucose trends right on your wrist.

SUMMARY: WHAT THE APPLE WATCH *CAN* AND *CANNOT* DO

Function	Apple Watch Alone	With CGM (e.g., Dexcom G7)
Measure blood sugar directly (non-invasive)	Cannot—Not FDA-approved	N/A
Display real-time glucose readings	N/A	Yes
Show glucose trends and alerts on the wrist	N/A	Yes
Help manage diabetes (with accurate data)	Dangerous if based on false readings	Effective with CGM support

Key Takeaway

- **Don't rely on your Apple Watch alone** to measure blood sugar—that's not safe or accurate.
- **Use it as a display device** when paired with an FDA-approved CGM, like the Dexcom G7 or FreeStyle Libre. That way, you get real-time glucose insights right on your wrist.

Stem Cells & Diabetes: The Future of Healing

WHAT ARE STEM CELLS?

- Stem cells are the body's **"master cells"** — they can turn into many different types of cells (like muscle, nerve, or pancreatic cells).
- For diabetes, the focus is on creating new **beta cells** (the cells in the pancreas that produce insulin).

TYPE 1 DIABETES & STEM CELLS

- In Type 1, the immune system attacks and destroys beta cells.
- Stem cell research aims to **replace or regenerate** these lost beta cells.
- Current clinical trials:
  - **Vertex Pharmaceuticals**: successfully implanted stem-cell–derived insulin-producing cells into Type 1 patients → some reduced or even eliminated the need for insulin injections.
  - **Encapsulation technology:** Protects new beta cells in a tiny "pouch" so the immune system can't destroy them.

TYPE 2 DIABETES & STEM CELLS

- In Type 2, the pancreas still makes insulin, but the body resists it. Over time, beta cells get "burned out."
- Stem cell therapy could:
  - Replace worn-out beta cells.
  - Reboot the pancreas function.
  - Support reversal in advanced cases.

TYPE 3 DIABETES (BRAIN CONNECTION)

- Stem cells aren't just for the pancreas. Researchers are exploring:
  - **Neural stem cells** → repair brain damage from Alzheimer's.
  - **Mesenchymal stem cells (MSCs)** → reduce inflammation, protect neurons.
- Early trials suggest MSCs may improve **memory and cognition** in dementia — potentially life-changing for the Type 3 link.

Challenges & Cautions

- **Immune rejection:** In Type 1, new cells may still be attacked unless protected.
- **Cost & access:** Still experimental, very expensive.
- **Regulation:** Only certain clinical trials are approved; beware of unregulated "stem cell clinics."
- **Long-term safety:** Researchers are still studying stability, cancer risk, and durability.

Hope for the Future

- Just like insulin changed diabetes 100 years ago, stem cells may offer a **functional cure** in the coming decades.
- For now, it's a developing therapy, not a treatment available to everyone.
- The takeaway for readers: **support your body now with lifestyle and holistic care**, while science advances toward regenerative medicine.

Key Takeaway:
Stem cell therapy represents the **cutting edge of diabetes care.** While not ready for everyday use, it offers real hope —

especially for **Type 1 (replacing destroyed beta cells)** and **Type 3 (repairing brain damage).**

Emerging & Future Therapies for Diabetes

1. GENE EDITING (CRISPR TECHNOLOGY)

- Scientists are experimenting with **CRISPR-Cas9** to correct genetic defects that lead to Type 1 or severe Type 2 diabetes.
- Goal: either stop the immune attack (Type 1) or restore insulin sensitivity (Type 2).
- Early lab results are promising, but human trials are still limited.

2. "SMART INSULIN" (GLUCOSE-RESPONSIVE INSULIN)

- Insulin that "turns on" only when blood sugar is high, then shuts off when sugar is normal.
- Would prevent dangerous lows (hypoglycemia).
- Several biotech companies are in **clinical testing** — which may reduce the need for constant monitoring.

3. PANCREATIC ISLET CELL TRANSPLANTS

- In Type 1, donor islet cells are transplanted into the liver, where they start making insulin.
- Some patients achieve **years of insulin independence.**
- Challenges: shortage of donor cells + need for immune-suppressing drugs.
- Stem cell–derived islets (like Vertex's trial) may solve the donor shortage.

4. ARTIFICIAL PANCREAS / CLOSED-LOOP SYSTEMS

- Combines **Continuous Glucose Monitor (CGM)** + **Insulin Pump** + AI algorithm.
- Automatically adjusts insulin based on real-time blood sugar.
- Already approved in many countries, with newer versions getting smarter (less manual input, more "hands-off").

5. KETONE & BRAIN-FUEL RESEARCH (TYPE 3 DIABETES LINK)

- Since the diabetic brain struggles to use glucose, researchers are studying **ketones (from ketogenic diets or MCT oil)** as an alternate brain fuel.
- Early results show improved memory and reduced Alzheimer's progression in some patients.
- Still debated: long-term safety of strict keto diets for all people with diabetes.

6. MICROBIOME THERAPY

- Gut bacteria strongly affect insulin resistance and cravings.
- Fecal microbiota transplants (FMT) are being studied to reset the microbiome in Type 2.
- Probiotic blends (with Akkermansia, Bifidobacterium) show promise in lowering blood sugar.

7. ANTI-INFLAMMATORY & IMMUNE THERAPIES

- Since inflammation drives both Type 2 and Type 3 diabetes, therapies target immune pathways:
  - **GLP-1 receptor agonists** (Ozempic, Mounjaro) → already widely used for sugar + weight.

    o **Anti-inflammatory drugs** like IL-1 blockers are being tested to protect beta cells in early Type 1.

8. NANOTECHNOLOGY & SENSORS

- Non-invasive glucose monitoring (like the dream Apple Watch sensor) → still under development.
- Nanoparticles that deliver insulin only where needed → in animal studies.
- Skin patches that painlessly release insulin or GLP-1 drugs → early trials.

9. REGENERATIVE MEDICINE BEYOND STEM CELLS

- **3D bioprinting of pancreas tissue** → experimental but could someday create replacement organs.
- **Peptide therapies** → molecules that encourage the body to repair beta cells naturally.

10. CHRONOTHERAPY (TIMING MEDICINE)

- Research shows that *when* you take insulin, eat carbs, or exercise, it may matter as much as *how much.*
- Aligning treatment with **circadian rhythms** could reduce complications.

Key Takeaway for Readers:
We're living in an era where diabetes treatment is shifting from **managing symptoms** to **seeking functional cures.** Stem cells, gene editing, artificial pancreas systems, microbiome resets, and even brain-fuel therapies are all in development. While not available to everyone yet, these breakthroughs mean the future of diabetes care looks more hopeful than ever.

Bibliography

MEDICAL & SCIENTIFIC SOURCES

- American Diabetes Association. (2023). *Standards of Medical Care in Diabetes—2023.* Diabetes Care, 46(Suppl. 1), S1–S290.
- De la Monte, S. M., & Wands, J. R. (2008). Alzheimer's disease is type 3 diabetes–evidence reviewed. *Journal of Diabetes Science and Technology,* 2(6), 1101–1113.
- Craft, S. (2005). Insulin resistance syndrome and Alzheimer's disease: Age- and obesity-related effects on memory, amyloid, and inflammation. *Neurobiology of Aging,* 26(1), 65–69.
- Holscher, C. (2019). Insulin signaling impairment in the brain as a risk factor in Alzheimer's disease. *Frontiers in Aging Neuroscience,* 11, 88.

NUTRITION & LIFESTYLE

- Fung, J. (2016). *The Obesity Code: Unlocking the Secrets of Weight Loss.* Greystone Books.
- Hyman, M. (2020). *The Blood Sugar Solution: 10-Day Detox Diet.* Little, Brown Spark.
- Perlmutter, D., & Colman, C. (2013). *Grain Brain: The Surprising Truth About Wheat, Carbs, and Sugar—Your Brain's Silent Killers.* Little, Brown and Company.
- Mosconi, L. (2018). *Brain Food: The Surprising Science of Eating for Cognitive Power.* Avery.

HERBAL & COMPLEMENTARY THERAPIES

- Balch, P. A. (2010). *Prescription for Herbal Healing.* Avery.
- Gladstar, R. (2012). *Herbal Recipes for Vibrant Health.* Storey Publishing.
- Bone, K., & Mills, S. (2013). *Principles and Practice of Phytotherapy: Modern Herbal Medicine.* Elsevier Health Sciences.

MIND-BODY & SPIRITUAL HEALING

- Hay, L. (1984). *You Can Heal Your Life.* Hay House.
- Chopra, D. (2009). *Reinventing the Body, Resurrecting the Soul.* Harmony Books.
- Kabat-Zinn, J. (2013). *Full Catastrophe Living: Using the Wisdom of Your Body and Mind to Face Stress, Pain, and Illness.* Bantam.

RESEARCH ON LIFESTYLE & PREVENTION

- Pan, X. R., et al. (1997). Effects of diet and exercise in preventing NIDDM in people with impaired glucose tolerance. *The Da Qing IGT and Diabetes Study.* Diabetes Care, 20(4), 537–544.
- Tuomilehto, J., et al. (2001). Prevention of type 2 diabetes mellitus by changes in lifestyle among subjects with impaired glucose tolerance. *The New England Journal of Medicine,* 344(18), 1343–1350.
- Knowler, W. C., et al. (2002). Reduction in the incidence of type 2 diabetes with lifestyle intervention or metformin. *The New England Journal of Medicine,* 346(6), 393–403.

Message From The Author

When I first began experiencing strange symptoms — the dreams, the trembling, the exhaustion, the fog — I didn't realize my body was speaking to me in its own urgent language. For years, I brushed it off, thinking I was simply tired, stressed, or "just getting older." But eventually, the truth revealed itself: my blood sugar was out of balance, and my brain and body were calling for help.

Writing this book has been both a healing and humbling journey. I've learned that Type 2 and Type 3 diabetes are not just about numbers on a lab sheet — they are about our relationship with food, with stress, with sleep, with joy, and most of all, with ourselves.

If you are holding this book in your hands, I want you to know this: **you are not alone.** The confusion, the cravings, the restless nights — they do not define you. They are simply messages, asking you to slow down, to listen, and to bring balance back into your life.

My deepest hope is that the tools, stories, and insights within these pages help you see your own path more clearly. That you discover not only how to stabilize blood sugar and protect your brain, but also how to rediscover the true sweetness of life — the kind found in connection, laughter, creativity, faith, and love.

Healing is not about perfection. It's about presence. It's about choosing one small step each day, and trusting that those steps add up to transformation.

From my heart to yours: may you walk this journey with courage, may you feel supported every step of the way, and may you never forget that your story is still unfolding — and it can be a story of health, joy, and renewal.

With love and faith in your healing,
Dr. Constance Santego

About the Author

Dr. Constance Santego, Ph.D., DNM, is a natural medicine doctor, educator, and author with over 25 years of experience in holistic healing, wellness education, and energy medicine. She is the founder of accredited wellness and esthetics programs in Canada and has trained thousands of students worldwide in modalities ranging from Reiki and reflexology to aromatherapy, massage therapy, and intuitive development.

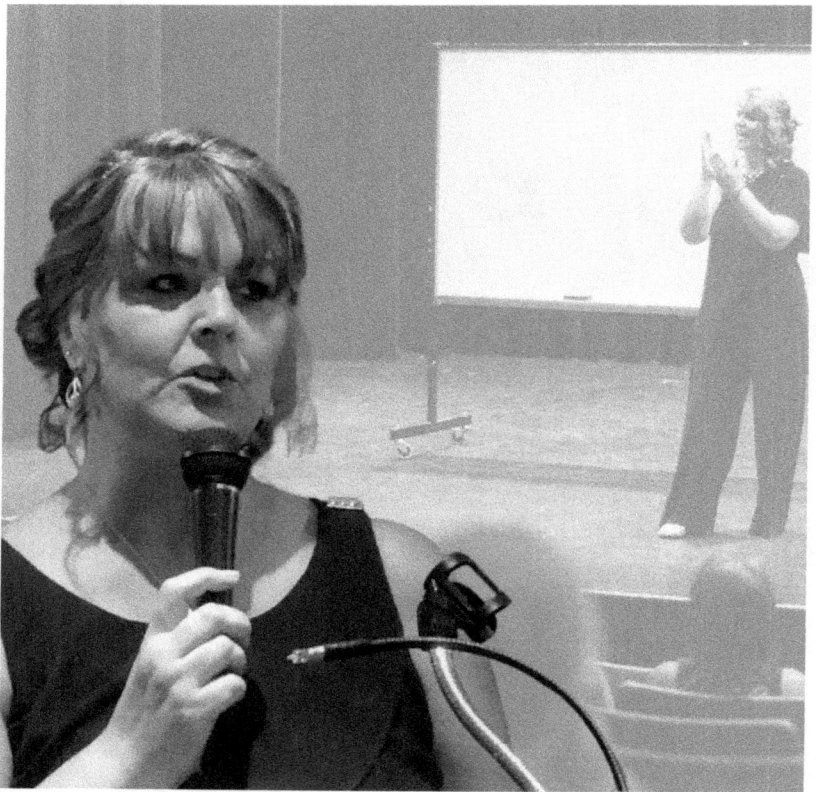

Her own journey with blood sugar imbalance and vivid nighttime "episodes" led her to explore the link between diabetes and brain health, often referred to as **Type 3 Diabetes.** This book was born from both personal experience and years of research, blending science, practical tools, and holistic wisdom.

Constance has authored more than 40 books across both fiction and nonfiction, including her **Reiki Wisdom Series**, *Secrets of a Healer* manuals, and inspirational novels rooted in spiritual growth. Her work bridges traditional medicine with complementary approaches, making complex ideas accessible and practical for everyday readers.

She is passionate about helping people discover that true healing is not only about managing symptoms, but about reclaiming **the sweetness of life** through balance, clarity, and joy.

When she's not writing or teaching, Constance enjoys life in beautiful British Columbia with her husband, surrounded by nature's calm and inspiration.

ALSO AVAILABLE

For additional information on

Constance Santego's

wide range of Motivational Products, Coaching Sessions,
Spiritual Retreats,
Live Events and Educational Programs

Go to

www.ConstanceSantego.ca

Follow on Instagram - Constance_Santego and
Facebook - constancesantegoo

Subscribe and receive Free Information and Meditations
on her
YouTube Channel - Constance Santego